CANCER PREV

CANCER FACTORS, CANCER FIGHTING FOODS AND HOW THE THREE SPICES – TURMERIC, GINGER AND GARLIC CAN REDUCE CANCER RISK.

JOSEPH VEEBE

Copyright © 2017 by Joseph Veebe. All Rights Reserved.

ISBN: 9781522082309

No part of this publication may be reproduced, distributed, or transmitted in any form or by any means, including photocopying, recording, or other electronic or mechanical methods, or by any information storage and retrieval system without the prior written permission of the publisher, except in the case of very brief quotations embodied in critical reviews and certain other noncommercial uses permitted by copyright law.

Cancer Prevention

Books in this Series:

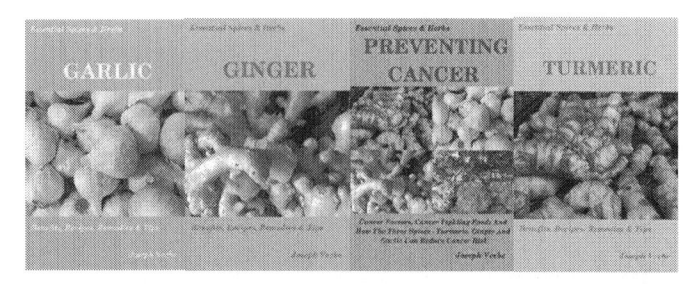

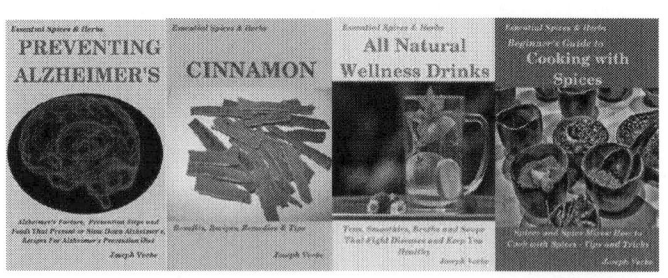

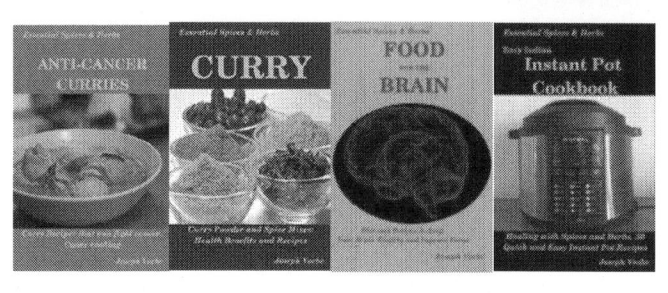

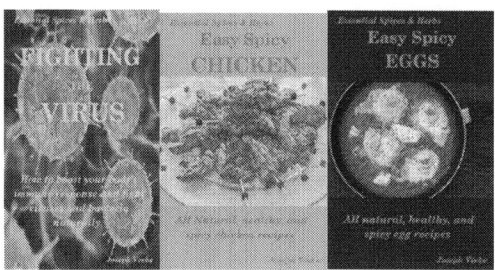

WHY I WROTE THIS BOOK

Cancer is a group of diseases characterized by the development of abnormal cells that multiply uncontrollably. These cancer cells then infiltrate normal body tissues and vital organs and impact their normal function, ultimately resulting in death. Cancer has the ability to spread throughout the body over a short period of time (often months or a couple of years). Cancer is caused by both external factors (chemicals, radiation, smoking, and infections) and internal factors (genetics, immune conditions, and hormones).

Cancer is the second leading cause of death in the United States. While there is no cure for many types of cancers, there has been significant progress in research and experimental treatments. More importantly, there have been more cancer awareness programs with an emphasis on prevention. It is estimated that more than half of all new cancers and cancer deaths are preventable by controlling the external or internal factors.

Many of us have heard that spices and herbs are good for health, but we hardly incorporate them into western cuisine. Even though there has been more awareness lately on the health benefits of herbs/spices as part of natural alternative or supplement to medicines, very few regularly incorporate spices and herbs in their diet. Some people hit nutritional stores to get natural supplements. While supplements are good, getting the same through natural foods is definitely preferable and can offer many nutrients that are not simply available in supplements.

Cancer Prevention

Lately, more and more studies have been conducted on health benefits spices, herbs, and other natural, unprocessed foods. These studies have shown that natural foods, herbs, and spices are effective in preventing and treating many modern debilitating diseases such as cancer, heart diseases, and Alzheimer's.

This book focuses on factors causing cancer and prevention, through a proper diet, including foods that help in preventing cancer and recipes to help prepare them. While there are many foods that are known to have positive effects on cancer prevention, the focus of this book is three essential spices – turmeric, ginger, and garlic, common ingredients in many food preparations. By liberally using these ingredients in cooking, many dishes can easily be transformed into cancer-fighting meals.

I have always loved cooking and always used spices in cooking due to my Asian heritage. But recently, I have started studying the many benefits of using spices and natural ingredients in food preparation. A healthy lifestyle can ward off many diseases and improve the quality of life for you and everyone around you. While I am a full convert to healthy living and lifestyle, I am hoping these books will inspire my children to live a healthy lifestyle at some point in their lives.

The lives of a number of my friends and colleagues have been impacted by cancer. This book is dedicated to their memory.

Cancer Prevention

TABLE OF CONTENTS

Why I Wrote This Book 3
Table of Contents 5
Chapter 1. Cancer Statistics 11
Chapter 2. Introduction & history of ginger, garlic, and turmeric 15
    Introduction 15
    History 16
    Turmeric – the golden spice 18
    Ginger – the tonic root 19
    Garlic – the stinking onion 20
Chapter 3. Cancer causing factors & how to avoid them 22
    Tobacco 22
    Alcohol 22
    Overweight 23
    Exercise and physical activity 23
    Radiation 23
    UV light 24
    Occupation 24
    Red meat and processed foods 24
    Fruits and vegetables 25
    Fiber 25
    Infections 25
    Other factors and tips to avoid cancer 26
Chapter 4. Cancer Fighting Foods 31
    Cancer fighter #1: Cruciferous Vegetables 31

| Cancer Prevention

Cancer fighter #2: Berries 32

Cancer Fighter #3: Nuts and Seeds 33

Cancer Fighter #4: Leafy Greens 35

Cancer Fighter #5: Tea 36

Cancer Fighter #6: Healthy Unrefined Oils 37

Cancer Fighter #7: Mushrooms 38

Cancer Fighter #8: Colorful Fruits and Veggies 40

Cancer Fighter#9: Healthy Protein: Wild Caught Fish, Organic Meats, Beans, Legumes, and Lentils 41

Cancer Fighter#10: Fermented Foods 42

Cancer Fighter#11: Spices & Herbs 44

Chapter 5. Anti-Cancer Properties of Turmeric, Ginger, and Garlic 45

    Anti-cancer properties 45

    Anti-oxidant properties 47

    Anti-inflammatory benefits 48

    Immune system and Infections 49

Chapter 6. Other Health Benefits of Turmeric, Ginger & Garlic 51

    Arthritis 52

    Neuro-protective 52

    Cholesterol 53

    Pain 54

    Improved circulation 54

    Anti-depressant 54

    Gastro-intestinal benefits 55

Skin and hair 55
Indigestion 56
Nausea and Morning Sickness 56
Diabetes and Heart Health 56
Lower blood pressure 57
Improved physical performance 57
Cold and Flu 57
Bone health 58
Antibacterial and anti-parasitic 58
Removing splinters 58
Detox agent 58

Chapter 7. Recipes with the cancer fighting trio of spices – turmeric, ginger & garlic 59

General tips for using turmeric, ginger, and garlic 59

Drinks 60

Basic turmeric tea 60
Basic ginger tea 62
Basic Mushroom Tea 62
Black tea with ginger and cardamom 63
Turmeric tea with ginger 64
Hot turmeric milk 65
Green tea with turmeric & ginger 66
Masala chai (spiced tea) 67
Ginger and lemon tea 68
Ginger ale 69
Tropical smoothie 70

Cancer Prevention

Green smoothie with garlic, ginger, and turmeric............71

Golden yellow smoothie 72

Very berry smoothie 72

Garlic drink with apple cider vinegar, lime, and honey .72

Garlic tea with ginger and lemon 73

Red wine and garlic 75

Garlic and lemon drink...76

Yogurt with turmeric, ginger, and garlic or yogurt curry
....77

Entrées and other dishes 78

Kale chips..78

Spinach/Red chard stir fry 79

Salmon with green mango..79

Broccoli stir fry..82

Bell pepper and chicken stir fry.......................................83

Coconut curry chicken 85

Cauliflower and potato..87

Tomato rice..89

Beef/Chicken pepper fry..90

Grilled chicken 91

Kale and chicken fry 94

Chapter 8. Tips For Buying & Using Turmeric, Ginger & Garlic 96

Buying..96

Cooking 96

Raw turmeric Vs. turmeric powder 97

| Cancer Prevention

    Ginger and garlic powders 97

    Ginger paste 98

    Garlic paste 98

        Ginger, garlic and turmeric paste 98

    Garlic oil 99

    Dosage 99

    Supplements 100

Chapter 9. Summary 101

    Disclaimer 106

Appendix I. Sources & References 108

    Cancer 108

    Hypertension 110

    Cholesterol & Blood Pressure 111

    Cold & Flu 112

    Detox 113

    Pain 113

    Arthritis 113

    Infections 113

    Diabetes & Blood Sugar 114

    Neuroprotective Properties 114

    Turmeric and Circulation 114

    Anti-inflammatory 114

    Cancer Statistics 114

Appendix II: Complete nutritional profile for turmeric, ginger & garlic 116

Appendix III. Home remedies using ginger, garlic and turmeric 122

    Ginger 122

    Garlic 122

    Turmeric 124

Preview of Other Books in this Series 125

    Essential Spices and Herbs: Turmeric 125

    Preventing Cancer 126

    Preventing Alzheimer's 127

    All Natural Wellness Drinks 129

    Essential Spices and Herbs: Ginger 129

    Essential Spices and Herbs: Garlic 130

    Essential Spices and Herbs: Cinnamon 131

    Anti-Cancer Curries 131

    Beginners Guide to Cooking with Spices 132

    Easy Indian Instant Pot Cookbook 133

    Fighting the Virus: How to Boost Your Body's Immune Response and Fight Virus Naturally 133

    Easy Spicy Eggs: All Natural Easy and Spicy Egg Recipes 134

    Food for the Brain 135

CHAPTER 1. CANCER STATISTICS

There were 14 million new cancer cases and 8.2 million cancer-related deaths in 2012 as per the World Health Organization (WHO). It is estimated that these figures will grow to 22 million new cancer cases and 13 million cancer-related deaths by 2030. Today, cancer is one of the most dreadful diseases facing humankind.

A recent report (12 September 2018) from the International Agency for Research on Cancer states that by the end of this century, cancer will be the number one killer in the world. Almost 10 million people will die of cancer this year (2018) and almost 18 million new cases. About one in five men and one in six women will develop cancer in their lifetimes.

In the United States, the estimate is about 1.7 million new cancer cases in 2017. Prostate cancer is the most common among males and breast cancer most common among females. It is estimated that there will be about 600,000 cancer-related deaths in 2017 in the USA.

The following table shows the incidence rate for various types of cancers in the US:

Cancer Prevention

Estimated New Cancer Cases in the US in 2017 (source ACS)			
Males - 836,000		Females - 853,000	
Prostate	19%	Breast	30%
Lung & bronchus	14%	Lung & bronchus	12%
Colon & rectum	9%	Colon & rectum	8%
Urinary bladder	7%	Uterine corpus	7%
Melanoma	6%	Thyroid	5%
Kidney &renal pelvis	5%	Melanoma	4%
Non-Hodgkin lymphoma	5%	Non-Hodgkin lymphoma	4%
Leukemia	4%	Leukemia	3%
Oral cavity &pharynx	4%	Pancreas	3%
Liver	3%	Kidney &renal pelvis	3%
All other types	23%	All other types	22%

The lifetime risk of developing cancer varies by country. For the United States, the lifetime risk for males is about 41%, a little less than 1 in 2. For U.S. females, the risk is 37%, a little more than 1 in 3. This percentage of risk is based on the entire population and depends on a number of external, internal, and lifestyle factors. For example, someone who follows a healthy lifestyle may have a significantly lower risk than someone who is overweight, smoker, and consumes processed foods and lead a sedentary lifestyle.

Cancer incidence rates worldwide vary by country and region. Africa, South East Asia, and China have one of the lowest rates of cancer incidence while North America (the US and Canada), Western Europe, and Australia have the highest incidence rates – in some cases as much as 3 times more than some of the Asian or African countries.

The following chart shows the incidence rate per 100,000 in the USA among various ethnic groups (data source: American Cancer Society).

Cancer Prevention

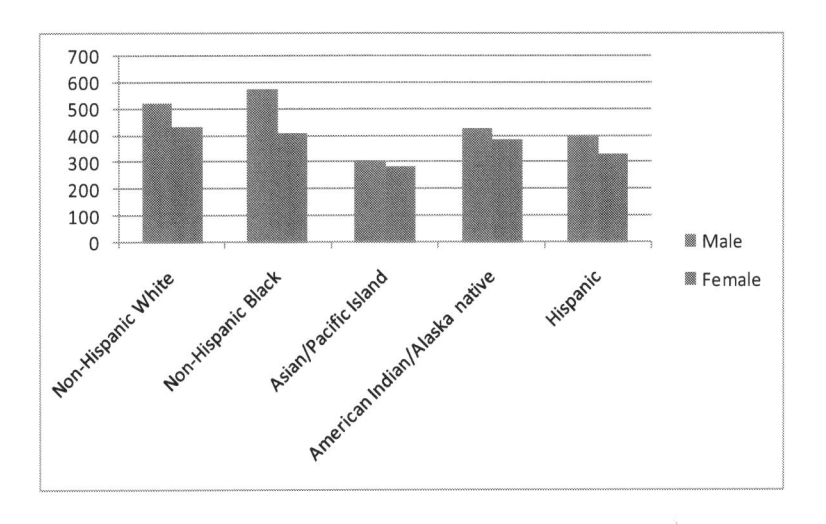

When one looks closely at worldwide cancer incidence data, it is clear that many developed countries have higher cancer rates than the developing or third world countries. There could be many factors causing this phenomenon, including industrialization, the use of chemicals in households and personal care, stress levels, and the use of more pre-prepared and processed foods than fresh meals.

A close examination of US cancer incidence data among various ethnic profiles also shows an interesting trend: Asians and Pacific Islanders almost have half the incident rate compared to white or black Americans. This shows that within the same country, lifestyles may have a significant impact on cancer incidence rates. Asians eat less processed meat and often go for a plant-based diet, using spices and herbs as part of food preparation. This author strongly believes food preparation and the use of spices and herbs is the differentiator in lower cancer incidence rates among Asians in the US.

Cancer is estimated to have the biggest economic impact among the many diseases worldwide. In 2006, medical costs for cancer care for the US were about $104.1 billion. As per estimate from the World Health Organization (WHO), the cost of premature death and disability from cancer was $895 billion worldwide compared to $753 billion for heart disease. This estimate does not include direct medical costs. The author estimates that the overall cost due to cancer, both care, and premature death and disability is well over a trillion dollars in 2017 worldwide (the author has not found any reliable estimates at the time of this writing).

Given the huge economic impact, major suffering to all the people involved – patients, family and caregivers – and the fact that there has not been any proper cure yet, we must do our best to promote prevention. The author believes that the easiest and most effective way of preventing and reducing the risk of cancer is through bettering your diet.

CHAPTER 2. INTRODUCTION & HISTORY OF GINGER, GARLIC, AND TURMERIC

INTRODUCTION

I want to thank you for purchasing this book, "Preventing Cancer". The book contains a lot of information about foods that help fight cancer, especially the three spices turmeric, ginger, and garlic. These spices have been used for several thousands of years both as medicine and as food flavoring ingredients.

Some of the spices used in modern times have been known to ancient civilizations and their health benefits are proven over thousands of years of use. Modern medicine has been increasingly studying many of these herbs and spices. However, there are many more organized studies are needed to get approval from the regulatory agencies for these herbs and spices to be accepted as part of mainstream prevention or treatment options for a number of medical conditions.

In this day and age of 'superfoods', organic foods, and healthy cooking and eating, the use of spices and herbs can be neglected.

We all want to eat healthy and tasty food. But we are all too busy to make fresh food at home. So, we settle for fast foods or packaged foods instead of healthy, homemade foods. The recipes listed in this book are quick and easy. The average time to cook is about 20 minutes.

Cancer Prevention

The book details the three spices turmeric, ginger, and garlic that are known and studied to have beneficial effects on cancer. All three of these spices are extremely beneficial to a healthy lifestyle. The book details many benefits of these ingredients. There are several recipes that readers can follow to incorporate these into one's daily food. The recipes are put together so that they can be easily prepared using common ingredients. There are several optional ingredients that you can try out to make the dish according to your personal taste and creativity.

This book also includes an extensive list of foods that help fight cancer. By arming oneself with the knowledge that many kinds of fruits, vegetables, and meats that are good for one's health and have been studied as potential cancer-preventing foods, one can modify their lifestyle/food habits to get maximum benefits out of this book.

HISTORY

Humans have used spices from the beginning of time. One can find references to various spices in ancient scripts such as the Old Testament, Bhagavad-Gita, and other writings. Ancient Egyptians, Chinese, Indians, Arabs, Greeks, and Romans have all used spices for various purposes, from cooking to food preservation and as medicine. There were many things that attracted humans to the use of spices – their aroma, their distinct taste, and their ability to flavor food, their color, and last but not the least, their medicinal properties. Archaeologists discovered the use of spices as preservatives or offerings in ancient Egyptian tombs and in other excavations. There are records of many civilizations around the world using herbs and spices for common ailments such as wound healing, fever, microbial infections, and more.

Garlic is believed to have originated in Central/West Asia. Ancient Indians have used it about 6000 years ago for its medicinal and aphrodisiac properties. Over the next thousand years, it spread to middle-east and Egypt to the Babylonian and Assyrian empires. Garlic was used in ancient times as a food seasoning and as a remedy for many common ailments. Romans and Egyptians fed garlic to warriors and slaves as it was believed to improve their strength. Garlic was also believed to ward off evil spirits, bring good luck, etc. People hung garlic in front of their homes as protection and seafarers carried garlic to prevent their ships from sinking in the sea. In medieval times, garlic was considered a remedy for plague and smallpox.

Unlike other spices, garlic always had a stigma, which may have arisen due to its pungent odor. It was believed to have aphrodisiac properties and even magical powers.

Americans started warming up to garlic since the 1940s as more and more of its benefits became known. Garlic consumption in America has tripled over the past decade or so. About 20 million tons of garlic produced in the world with more than half coming out of China.

Similar to turmeric and garlic, ginger use also dates back from 4000 to5000 years by Indians and Chinese. Indians used ginger as a standalone flavoring ingredient in drinks such as buttermilk and ginger teas. Ginger was used in Ayurvedic medicine as a substance that helped with stomach ailments and nausea. Ginger was often used in conjunction with garlic and turmeric (in paste form) to flavor curries in Indian cuisine.

In summary, all three of these spices have been used for over 4000 years by ancient Indians, Chinese, and Egyptians in conjunction or individually and have a rich history. There is some evidence that the Indus Valley civilization which was at its peak about 2500 BC used all three spices – turmeric, ginger, and garlic. Turmeric was also used as an important part of Ayurvedic medicine for wound healing and treating infections.

TURMERIC – THE GOLDEN SPICE

Turmeric is a well-known spice in Asian cooking, especially South Asia. Turmeric comes from the root of the turmeric plant which is part of the ginger family. The turmeric root is cleaned, dried, and grinded to create the yellow turmeric powder. Turmeric is used as an herbal supplement, added to flavor food as part of curry powder or as a standalone spice, added to cosmetics, or used as a food coloring. Turmeric is also used as a skin treatment and beauty enhancer. Evidently, it has been used by humans for thousands of years and is a time-tested wonder. This chapter will focus on turmeric and its benefits as part of food and cooking.

Turmeric powder is bright yellow and provides the distinct yellow color to the Indian "curry powder." Turmeric has been one of the key ingredients in Asian cuisine for years.

The main active ingredient in turmeric is called curcumin, which has very powerful medicinal properties. However, there are two challenges in fully realizing the benefits of turmeric.

One, the curcumin content is only about 3% of turmeric by weight. Second, curcumin is not easily absorbed by the body. Curcumin absorption can be substantially enhanced by consuming black pepper which contains piperine along with turmeric. Also, fatty foods have been proven to aid curcumin absorption as well. To consume a sufficient dosage of curcumin, a combination of curcumin/turmeric extract supplements along with a diet prepared with turmeric is recommended.

Turmeric is a rich source of many essential vitamins and minerals; it does not contain any cholesterol but is an excellent source of antioxidants and dietary fiber which helps to control bad cholesterol levels.

Fresh turmeric root is a very good source of several vitamins such as vitamin-C, vitamin B-6, vitamin-E, and niacin. Turmeric is also a great source of minerals such as calcium, iron, potassium, manganese, copper, zinc, and magnesium.

Turmeric's antioxidant levels are one of the highest among popular spices and herbs. An in-depth nutritional profile for turmeric is in the table in appendix ii.

GINGER – THE TONIC ROOT

Ginger (*Zingiber officinale*) is a flowering plant whose root is widely used as a spice and traditional medicine over thousands of years in Asia. Ginger belongs to the same family as turmeric and cardamom.

Ginger is widely used in Asian cooking, especially China and India. While turmeric, which belongs to the same family as ginger is mostly used in the powder form, ginger is used as a fresh ingredient in most cooking.

Ginger has been one of the key ingredients in Asian cuisine for centuries, especially used as part of meat recipes. When dried and ground, ginger results in a white powder that is used in baking (gingerbread, cookies, crackers, cakes etc.) and making beverages (ginger ale, ginger beer, etc.). Ginger, either powdered or fresh, can be used in teas and is an essential component of 'masala chai'.

The main bioactive active ingredient in ginger is called gingerol and it has very powerful medicinal properties. Ginger is used in several alternative/traditional medicines in the East.

Unlike turmeric, ginger is not a significant source of vitamins and minerals. More than 75% of raw ginger is water. Ginger does contain small amounts of minerals and vitamins as in the table below. The most important component of ginger is gingerol which provides its anti-oxidant and anti-inflammatory properties.

GARLIC – THE STINKING ONION

Garlic is part of the *Allium* (onion) family and is closely related to shallots, onions, Chinese onions, chives, and leeks. There are 400+ varieties of garlic in the world today.

When one thinks of garlic, the first thing that comes to mind is the smell. But beyond its sharp odor, garlic offers a number of health benefits. While most garlic production and consumption is in Asia, garlic is finding more and more uses in the west in cooking and health supplements. China produces more than ½ of the world garlic production, close to

20 million tons. More than 90% of all garlic production in the USA comes out of California.

Most garlic bulbs are white in color and consist of 10 or more cloves. Garlic enhances the flavor of many dishes such as Indian curries, Chinese food, pizzas, and stir-fries.

The main active ingredient in garlic is called polysulphide allicin and is responsible primarily for its medicinal properties. This compound, allicin, formed when garlic cloves are chopped or crushed not only provides the medicinal properties but the distinct taste and smell as well.

Garlic is extremely nutritious and is a source of vitamins C and B6, along with the minerals manganese and selenium. Garlic also contains minor amounts of other minerals such as calcium, copper, potassium, phosphorous, and iron.

Just three cloves of garlic (about 9 grams) a day provides a recommended daily value of 8% manganese, 7 % vitamin B6, 4% vitamin C, 3% copper, 3 % selenium and 2% each phosphorous, calcium and vitamin B1.

Before we discuss the benefits of these three spices in the cancer-fighting regime, it is important for us to understand the factors causing cancer and how to avoid them.

CHAPTER 3. CANCER CAUSING FACTORS & HOW TO AVOID THEM

This chapter lists several factors that increase the risk of cancer. By consciously avoiding these wherever or whenever possible coupled with foods that help reduce such risk (discussed in the next chapter), one can significantly reduce the risk of getting cancer. It is to be noted that these steps only reduce the risk but do not completely eliminate the risk. I have met people who lived a healthy lifestyle and still were diagnosed with cancer. It only takes one cell in your body to go rogue and multiply but any steps that can reduce the risk are worth it.

TOBACCO

Tobacco is one of the biggest contributing factors to lung cancer. While people are becoming more aware of the risks of smoking or chewing tobacco, there are still a large number of people in the world who use tobacco. One should avoid tobacco in active or passive (second-hand smoke) form to help reduce the risk of lung or other related cancers.

ALCOHOL

While some studies suggest that moderate alcohol consumption is actually good, too much alcohol is believed to increase the risk of cancer. By cutting down alcohol and tracking the amount you drink, you can reduce the risk significantly.

OVERWEIGHT

Many people are not aware that being overweight increases the risk of cancer. Keeping a healthy weight can not only help improve one's quality of life but also significantly reduce the risk of cancer. American Cancer Society notes that being overweight accounts for 20% of cancer deaths in women and 14% in men. If you are overweight, make it a point to reduce your weight by at least 10 pounds.

EXERCISE AND PHYSICAL ACTIVITY

Being physically active not only helps to control the weight but also helps reduce the risk of cancer. One does not need to spend hours in the gym every day to get benefits; simply walking for 30 minutes a day, doing household chores, etc. get you the benefit. Even when you need to work at a desk or watch TV, standing up to work or watch TV will be more beneficial than sitting for a majority of the time. Even if you are not a fan of exercise, simply avoiding sitting down to work, watch tv or do chores can have immense health benefits including benefits that lead to preventing cancer.

RADIATION

While we are all exposed to a certain amount of radiation all the time such as microwave, cell phone, electric lines, radio waves, etc., exposure to higher doses of radiation – such as close to electric transmission lines, microwave towers or even x-rays or radiation treatment, etc. can increase the risk of cancer. While some of these (for example an x-ray for a broken bone) may be unavoidable, be aware of the radiation surrounding you are in. Use hands-free devices on your cell phone whenever possible and avoid high transmission lines or unnecessary X-rays to help reduce the risk.

UV LIGHT

Getting too much UV light can increase the risk of cancer. Exposure to UV light could come from exposure to the sun or suntan spas. Melanoma and other skin cancers have a direct correlation to exposure from the sun's UV light or too many visits to tanning salons.

OCCUPATION

People who work in chemical factories or other places where there are harmful particles or smoke are at increased risk of cancer. You should take workplace safety seriously and follow all workplace safety rules (e.g. wearing masks). If you are not in a safe environment, work with the management to improve the safety for you and others.

RED MEAT AND PROCESSED FOODS

Red meats primarily include beef, lamb, pork, or any other animal meat such as deer, buffalo, etc.

Processed meats include any meat that has added preservatives or is processed to a different form such as salami, bacon, ham, sausages and others.

Processed foods most often contain harmful chemicals as preservatives or other food additives.

One does not have to completely avoid these foods. However, limiting the intake and being conscious about their harmful effects is a good start.

FRUITS AND VEGETABLES

As you have seen from the previous chapter, many fruits and vegetables contain cancer-fighting compounds, and consuming them on a daily basis in the recommended 5 servings provides you significant health benefits including reducing the risk of cancer. However, many people eat fewer than the recommended amount, which is critical to increased wellbeing.

FIBER

Intake of a high fiber diet helps the digestive system by helping to speed up food passing through the digestive tract. This force cancer-causing chemicals in food to move through the body quickly and avoid absorption into the body. Fiber is known to reduce the risk specifically of bowel cancer.

INFECTIONS

Infections can cause certain types of cancers. For example, cervical cancer is linked with HPV or Human Papilloma Virus where virus DNA alters human DNA, resulting in abnormal cell growth. Similarly, the risk of stomach cancer increases as a result of infection with Helicobacter pylori (H pylori) bacteria.

OTHER FACTORS AND TIPS TO AVOID CANCER

Salt

A diet high in salt can not only cause increased blood pressure but can also increase the risk of stomach cancer.

Hormone Replacement Therapies (HRT):

Hormone replacement therapy can potentially increase the risk of cancer.

Avoid bottled water and drink filtered tap water

If your tap water is filtered well, it is usually equal in quality to bottled water. Moreover, tap water is from a known source following standard/regulated municipal purification process, whereas sources of bottled water are unknown. In addition, plastic bottles could contain chemical compounds, such as BPA, that could contaminate the water. Filtering tap water to remove any harmful compounds may be more beneficial than the regular consumption of bottled water.

Walk at least 30 minutes a day

Physical activity is a key to warding off many diseases including cancer, slow aging, slow down Alzheimer's, and many other neurodegenerative diseases. Studies have shown that walking at least 30 minutes a day lowers colon and breast cancer risk.

Breastfeeding

There have been some studies showing that breastfeeding helps ward off breast cancer. Thus, by breastfeeding, if one is able to, you can reduce the risk of breast cancer.

Get out of the chair/sofa. Stand more

Modern occupations and lifestyles result in people spending a lot of time sitting. If your work requires sitting at a desk, try to get a standing desk. Try to use your smartphone/watch to remind you to stand up after sitting for an hour or so. Stand up and watch TV instead of sitting down. One study showed that people who spent most of their time sitting had a 50% higher risk of colon cancer compared to people who sat less.

Eat healthy (see next chapter)

The next chapter describes many cancer-fighting foods. Some may think that eating healthy is expensive, but if you consider the long-term costs of unhealthy eating, healthy eating habits pays for itself in the longer term and enables you to have a more trouble free (from a health perspective) life.

Avoid microwaving plastic containers

Plastic containers could potentially have harmful BPA compounds. Microwaving could get these harmful chemicals into your food.

Include spices in your food (more garlic, turmeric, and ginger; see the chapter on recipes)

This is the focus of this book. See subsequent chapters on how including spices can help to reduce the risk of cancer.

Marinate meat before cooking

Some studies have shown that marinating meat before cooking helps block the creation of cancer-causing compounds called heterocyclic amines. These compounds could modify the DNA of cells to trigger tumor growth. Many of the meat recipes listed in this book include a step to marinate the meat before cooking using some of the antioxidant spices that protect against the formation of these compounds.

Drink teas (see the chapter on recipes)

Consumption of coffee and tea has been found to reduce the risk of various types of cancer. Green tea is especially rich in antioxidants and has great potential for fighting against cancer. The next chapter gives some more details on various kinds of teas and their benefits.

Avoid fatty protein

Eating too much red meat increases the risk of heart disease and cancer compared to people who do not eat meat or eat lean protein such as poultry or fish. Switch to a vegan protein such as lentils and beans, low fat or non-fat dairy, poultry, or fish instead of beef or other fatty meat.

Eat more onions

Foods in the onion family (garlic, red/yellow/white onions, shallots, scallions, chives) all have high anti-oxidant capabilities and natural compounds that prevent cell growth. Onions are highly effective cancer fighters and can be found in many of the recipes in this book.

Avoid fried foods

Frying food in oil at high temperatures results in a chemical called acrylamide forming in the food. This chemical has shown to increase the risk of cancer. Avoid French fries, potato chips, and other fried foods whenever you can.

Stop tanning

Several studies have shown that tanning increases the risk of skin cancer.

Avoid dry cleaning

Dry cleaners use a chemical called perc which has been shown to cause kidney and liver damage with repeated exposures.

Drink plenty of water

Drinking the recommended 8 glasses or more of water not only helps you stay hydrated but helps to dilute cancer causing substances in the urine, which reduces the risk of bladder cancer.

Avoid chemicals wherever possible – home cleaning, insecticides, lawn/garden chemicals, etc.

Anything that is harmful for another living thing is harmful for humans as well. So, insecticides, disinfectants, cleaning products, or other chemicals can harm you and possibly trigger cancer incidents. Look at the label before buying them. Organic, natural insecticides and cleaning products are probably less risky than the regular variety. One should especially be careful about using these around children. A recent California lawsuit against Roundup, a popular weed killer found that exposure to glyphosate, the main ingredient of the weed killer can cause cancer.

Eat whole grains and avoid white eats

Try to eat whole grains – whole wheat, whole oats, brown rice, whole-grain barley, quinoa, whole-grain cereal. Avoid white foods – white rice, white bread, white pasta, potatoes, white sugar, bleached flour, etc.

Avoid sodas or drink in moderation

Sodas have too many chemicals, sweeteners, and sugars that are not good for your health. Substitute water whenever possible. When you do crave soda, use smaller cans or smaller sizes.

Avoid combo meals / super-size at fast food places

Cut down your visits to fast food joints. Many fast foods have a lot of preservatives that could increase cancer risk or cause other health problems. When you do visit, avoid ordering combo meals but pick and choose what you want.

The next chapter discusses many foods that are known to fight and reduce the risk of cancer.

CHAPTER 4. CANCER FIGHTING FOODS

While the focus of this book is on the spices turmeric, ginger, and garlic, it is essential to understand other cancer-fighting foods and their specific benefits. By using these three spices and others as part of preparing meals out of these cancer fighting foods, we can achieve even better results in the fight against cancer.

CANCER FIGHTER #1: CRUCIFEROUS VEGETABLES

All cruciferous vegetables, such as broccoli, cauliflower, cabbage, and kale, are considered very good for fighting and preventing cancer. As per the American Institute for Cancer Research, they contain a compound called *sulforaphane*, which may boost the production of the body's protective enzymes and help flush out carcinogens. Besides *sulforaphane*, cruciferous vegetables also contain other cancer fighters such as *glucosinolates*, *crambene*, and *indole-3-carbinol*.

Broccoli is the most potent cancer fighter of all cruciferous vegetables.

The recommended list:

- Broccoli
- Kale
- Cauliflower
- Cabbage – all varieties (red, green, Chinese, Napa, etc.)
- Bok Choy

- Collard Greens

Cancers they may help fight:

- Breast cancer
- Liver cancer
- Lung cancer
- Prostate cancer
- Skin Cancers
- Cancers in the stomach
- Bladder cancers

Suggestions:
Use these vegetables in whichever way you can – sautéed, steamed, pizza or salads. I have included some recipes that combine the power of spices with kale, broccoli, and cauliflower.

CANCER FIGHTER #2: BERRIES

All berries are rich in antioxidants, which help neutralize free radicals in the body that usually cause cell damage. Cell damage is a pathway for many cancers and other diseases, along with aging.

The main phytochemicals in berries are called anthocyanins. These antioxidants can counteract, reduce, or slow down the growth of cancer cells and possibly prevent new blood vessels from forming in the cancerous cells. Berries are rich in other nutrients such as vitamin C, fiber, and minerals which can fight cancer in addition to the anti-oxidants.

Cancer Prevention

The recommended list:

- Blueberries
- Blackberries
- Raspberries
- Strawberries
- Acai berries
- Goji berries
- Cherries

Cancers they may fight:

- Skin Cancers
- Bladder cancer
- Lung cancer
- Breast cancer
- Esophageal cancer

Suggestions:
Eat them raw. Add them to smoothies or juice them. Makes sure to wash them thoroughly before eating as insecticides or other chemicals used in farming, preserving, or transporting are washed off as much as possible. Use organic versions when possible.

CANCER FIGHTER #3: NUTS AND SEEDS

If you have not incorporated nuts and seeds into your diet, you should seriously consider adding them. At least 2-3 handfuls of nuts and seeds a week will provide you with immense benefits.

While all nuts and seeds are healthy, walnuts, pecans, and flax seeds are especially good cancer fighters. Walnuts and pecans have been shown to block estrogen receptors in breast cancer cells, possibly slowing the growth of such cells. Nuts have also been shown to slow the growth of cancer cells in pancreatic and liver cancer patients.

Flax seeds contain lignans, which have antioxidants that are found to help in neutralizing or arresting the growth of cancer cells, especially in breast cancer. Flaxseed is also high in omega-3 fatty acids, which can protect against colon cancer and prevent heart disease.

The recommended list:

- Walnuts
- Pecans
- Almonds
- Brazil nuts
- Peanuts
- Cashews

Seeds:

- Flax seeds
- Chia seeds
- Hemp seeds
- Sunflower seeds
- Pumpkin seeds

Cancers they may help fight:

- Breast cancer
- Liver cancer
- Prostate cancer
- Pancreatic cancer

Suggestions:

Make it point to eat a handful of seeds/nuts every day. Replace your unhealthy snacks with nuts and seeds. Add them to smoothies. Top cereal bowls with nuts and berries. Snack on them instead of potato chips or other junk foods.

CANCER FIGHTER #4: LEAFY GREENS

Dark leafy green vegetables have been getting more and more attention lately for their health benefits. According to the American Institute of Cancer research, dark green leafy vegetables have a wide range of carotenoids such as *lutein* and *zeaxanthin*, along with saponins and flavonoids. Carotenoids prevent cancer by acting as antioxidants that lookout for potentially dangerous free radicals and neutralize them.

The recommended list:

Kale (all types – green, red, Lacinato)

- Spinach
- Chard
- Collard greens
- Mustard greens
- Dandelion greens

Cancers they may fight:

- Breast cancer
- Skin cancers
- Lung cancers
- Stomach cancer

- Mouth, pharynx and larynx cancers

Suggestions:
Make them part of smoothies and salads. Sauté those with onions, garlic, ginger, etc. Add some turmeric and coconut powder. Cream them or toss some chopped greens into your meat preparations.

CANCER FIGHTER #5: TEA

According to the National Cancer Institute, more than 60 studies have been conducted on the effects of regular tea consumption and the risk of cancer. While some of the results have been inconsistent, there is evidence that the consumption of tea reduced the risk of specific cancers such as cancers of colon, breast, ovary, prostate, and lung.

The antioxidant chemicals (catechins) in teas have the ability to scavenge for free radicals in the body and neutralize them. Of all the tea varieties, green tea offers the most promise as cancer fighting tea drink.

The recommended list:

- Green tea
- Black tea
- Chamomile tea
- Dandelion tea
- Essiac tea

Cancers they may fight:

- Breast cancer
- Colon cancer
- Ovarian cancer

- Prostate cancer
- Lung cancer

Suggestions:
Make a couple of cups of tea a day as part of your daily routine.

CANCER FIGHTER #6: HEALTHY UNREFINED OILS

Using unrefined oils such as coconut oil, extra virgin olive oil and cod oil instead of refined oil can help improve the immune system. They also have Omega-3 fatty acids that can help nourish the cells in your body and keep them healthy and prevent oxidation.

Cancers they may fight:

- Tongue cancer
- Colon cancer
- Breast cancer
- Skin cancers

Suggestions:
Use these unrefined oils for cooking.

Cancer Fighter #7: Mushrooms

Mushrooms have been used in eastern medicines for hundreds and possibly thousands of years. Mushrooms have been part of eastern cuisines for a long time as well.

Studies have been conducted regarding the ability of certain types of mushrooms to fight cancer. The main benefit of these anti-cancer mushrooms is their ability to enhance the body's immune system which fights and defends against many diseases including cancer. The main types of mushrooms that are believed to have anti-cancer properties are:

- Reishi mushrooms
- Maitake mushrooms
- Chaga mushroom
- Turkey Tail mushroom
- Shitake mushrooms
- Chinese Caterpillar fungus
- Agaricus Blazei mushrooms

These mushrooms have been researched and have been found to help fight cancer due to their immune-boosting and antioxidant capabilities. Some of these have even exhibited antiviral and tumor-shrinking capabilities. In some cases, a combination of multiple mushroom extracts has shown to provide cumulative and amplified benefits, as they work well together.

In some parts of the east (especially Japan), patients take mushroom extracts alongside chemotherapy for both maximum benefit and to reduce the side effects of cancer treatment.

Cancer Prevention

Cancers they may fight:

- Colon cancer
- Breast cancer
- Lung cancer
- Prostate cancer

Suggestions:
Mushrooms may be cooked as is or chopped and put in as part of other dishes, salads, pizza toppings, or eggs. Make mushrooms a part of your weekly diet.

Chaga mushroom is one of the more popular mushrooms used in the natural/supplemental treatment for cancer. Chaga mushrooms are found in the Northern hemisphere and is used in folk medicine for centuries. Chaga mushrooms have a lot of nutrients but recently researchers have been looking at potential benefits of Chaga mushrooms in preventing and slowing down its growth.

A study conducted in 2009 showed that a chemical compound found in Chaga and other mushrooms called *triterpenes* can help tumor cells to self-destruct while not harming healthy cells. A 2010 petri dish study found that Chaga mushroom could slow growth of lung, breast, and cervical cancer cells.

With its various properties chaga mushrooms could be used to stimulate immune system, reduce inflammation and prevent or treat cancer.

Chaga mushroom is edible but is bitter in taste. Best way to consume chaga mushroom is to make tea from chaga powder. Chaga mushroom should be avoided if you are on blood-thinning medications.

CANCER FIGHTER #8: COLORFUL FRUITS AND VEGGIES

One of the oft-made suggestions for healthy eating is the notion of "eating the colors of the rainbow." Brightly colored vegetables and fruits carry abundant phytochemicals that are full of carotenoid antioxidants and other essential vitamins.

Beta-carotene, one of the many carotenoids found in colored vegetables has been studied and found to have benefits in fighting cancers of eye, skin, and other vital organs in the body besides being helpful in detoxification and in boosting the immune system.

Below are some common fruits and vegetables that are colorful which should find a way into one's daily diet plans. Many of these foods have been shown to fight several cancers such as stomach, ovarian, breast and lung cancers.

Pink/Red – Tomatoes, watermelon, red chard, pomegranate, cherries, strawberries, apples, bell peppers, raspberries, and grapefruit.

Blue/Purple – Eggplant, grapes, beets, red cabbage, purple cauliflower, blueberries, and prunes.

Yellow/Orange – Orange, apricots, papaya, mango, banana, pineapple, carrot, pumpkins, and squash.

Green – Bright green leafy vegetables - kale, spinach, peppers, celery, and artichokes.

Cancers they may fight:

- Eye cancer

- Skin cancers
- Colon cancer
- Pancreatic cancer
- Ovarian cancer

Suggestions:
Make it a point to eat one or two servings of colored vegetables/fruits a day. Fruits may be part of smoothies; vegetables may be combined with other spices/herbs or eaten as part of a salad.

CANCER FIGHTER#9: HEALTHY PROTEIN: WILD CAUGHT FISH, ORGANIC MEATS, BEANS, LEGUMES, AND LENTILS

Protein is an important building block of the human body – bones, muscles, blood, skin, and cartilage all have proteins in them. Protein is used to build and repair tissues. It also makes important body chemicals such as enzymes and hormones, helps in improving metabolism and losing weight, and much more. It is recommended that one consume 1 gram of protein for every 3 lbs. of body weight.

Since protein is a macro-nutrient and is essential in your daily diet, one must eat healthy protein as part of your fight against cancer. Organic meats and wild-caught fish are devoid of any cancer-causing substances. They are also packed with vitamins and minerals (and omega-3 in the case of fish) besides offering clean protein.

If you want to avoid animal proteins, beans, lentils, and legumes offer a healthy alternative. Colored beans, especially black and navy beans, offer great protective benefits against colon cancer as they contain higher levels of fatty acid butyrate.

Cancers they may fight:

- Breast cancer
- Colon cancers

Suggestions:

Balance your protein intake with both animal and vegetable proteins. Add one serving of legumes/lentils into your meals 2-3 times a week. Soak dry legumes in water overnight and either cook it or toss it as part of a salad. While cooking, it is beneficial to add other spices (described in this book – turmeric, ginger, and garlic) to get the maximum defense against cancer.

CANCER FIGHTER#10: FERMENTED FOODS

There are trillions of microorganisms that live in our bodies. Most of them live in our gut or digestive system. These "good bacteria" living in our gut contribute to digestion, help improves immunity, and are hugely important to maintaining our health and our body's ability to fight disease.

Fermented foods are rich in probiotics and eating fermented food is a sure way to improve immunity and help digestion.

The recommended list:

- Yogurt – provides billions of probiotic cultures
- Kefir – fermented milk drink abundant in probiotics
- Kombucha - fermented tea
- Raw non-pasteurized cheese – provides active cultures
- Sauerkraut – made of fermented cabbage
- Kimchi – Korean version of sauerkraut; fermented vegetables including cabbage.
- Pickles – pickle anything and it is good for your gut
- Miso – made of fermented soybeans with barley/brown rice and koji. A traditional Japanese dish/seasoning
- Tempeh – a fermented soybean product; a traditional soybean product of Indonesia.

Cancers they may fight:

Consuming fermented foods with tons of "good bacteria" keeps our digestive system healthy, helps build immunity and enhances the overall cancer fighting capabilities of the body.

Suggestions:
Include 2-3 servings of one or more of these fermented foods in your diet a week.

Cancer Fighter #11: Spices & Herbs

There are a number of spices and herbs that have shown promise in fighting cancer. Three of them stand out. While there are many foods that have cancer fighting capabilities, by using turmeric, ginger, and garlic for seasoning, every meal or every drink becomes a meal or drink that helps in fighting cancer. The next chapter details the properties that make turmeric, ginger, and garlic super foods against cancer.

CHAPTER 5. ANTI-CANCER PROPERTIES OF TURMERIC, GINGER, AND GARLIC

In this chapter, we examine the trio of spices for their direct and indirect anti-cancer properties. Turmeric, garlic, and ginger are spices that have been used for thousands of years and as such are proven to be extremely safe for both their medicinal and culinary uses. They all contain excellent chemical compounds that provide direct benefits for specific cancers and indirect benefits due to specific properties such as anti-inflammatory, antioxidant, and immune boosting abilities. Let us examine these properties a bit closely:

ANTI-CANCER PROPERTIES

There have been more than a thousand studies conducted on the effects of curcumin, the active compound in turmeric, on cancer cells. These tests in the lab have shown that turmeric can kill or arrest the growth of cancer cells. Some studies on test animals have shown that turmeric blocked the formation of cancer-causing enzymes. Thus, turmeric could be used not only as a treatment but as prevention as well. Turmeric as part of a regular diet keeps your digestive system healthy and helps ward off colon cancer.

Many of the curcumin studies are focused on the benefits of curcumin in cancers such as colon, prostate, breast cancer and osteosarcoma.

Ginger contains the compound called 6-gingerol which is a very effective anticancer agent. 6-gingerol activates molecular mechanisms in the cancer cells that effectively destroys cells by causing them to commit suicide.

There have been many studies conducted on the effects of ginger in colorectal cancer patients that have shown the effectiveness of ginger in arresting the growth of cancer cells. This may not be surprising given how good ginger is for the gastrointestinal system. Ginger is believed to be also effective in other forms of cancer such as pancreatic cancer, ovarian cancer, and breast cancer. Further studies are required to confirm this.

Ginger's anti-nausea properties can help to treat nausea and vomiting caused by cancer treatment and chemotherapy.

There have been a number of studies conducted, especially in Asia, on the effectiveness of garlic against certain types of cancers. These studies, both the population and clinical, have shown the potential benefits of garlic in the stomach, colon, pancreas, esophagus, and breast cancers.

A couple of different population studies in China have shown the reduced risk of stomach, esophagus, and prostate cancers in a population taking garlic compared to a population not taking garlic.

A study in San Francisco showed a 50% lower pancreatic cancer risk for people taking a larger amount of garlic compared to people not taking garlic or taking lower amounts.

All three of the spices – turmeric, ginger, and garlic help reduce risks for many cancers individually and when used together can work in combination to potentially reduce the risk for a broad spectrum of cancers.

In the next sections, we will examine other properties of these three essential spices that provide complementary benefits to cancer fighting properties.

ANTI-OXIDANT PROPERTIES

Oxidative damage caused by free radicals (highly reactive molecules with unpaired electrons) contributes to the risk of cancers, heart disease, and diabetes as well as age-related macular degeneration. Free radicals tend to react with important organic substances, such as fatty acids, proteins, or DNA, causing oxidative damage.

Antioxidants help neutralize free radicals and reduce the risk of oxidative damage. They "clean up" free radicals by interacting and forming harmless substances, thereby protecting healthy cells. There are several vitamins and supplements that are known to have antioxidant properties (e.g. vitamin C & E, beta carotene, etc.). Many fruits (berries, grapes, etc.) and vegetables (kale, artichokes, bell pepper, etc.) contain antioxidants. Nuts such as walnuts and beverages such as tea and coffee also contain antioxidants. Antioxidants are often added to packaged food products to keep them from interacting with air.

Curcumin, the active ingredient in turmeric, is a potent antioxidant that can do two things: neutralize free radicals due to its chemical structure and stimulate the body's own antioxidant enzymes.

Cancer Prevention

Regular garlic intake has shown to increase antioxidant enzymes in the body especially in diabetics and patients of hypertension.

Once again, anti-oxidant foods help neutralize free radicals in the body that cause oxidative cell damage and potentially cause cancer and other debilitating diseases.

ANTI-INFLAMMATORY BENEFITS

Inflammation plays an important role in the natural healing process in the human body. It helps to defend harmful invaders in our body such as bacteria that cause infection. Inflammation also helps the body carry out wound repair. Without inflammation, foreign invaders could cause damage to our bodies and ultimately kill us.

When short term, controlled inflammation is beneficial. It can become a major problem when it becomes chronic, such as arthritis. Chronic inflammation plays a major role in many serious health conditions such as heart disease, cancer, Alzheimer's and other various degenerative conditions.

Therefore, it is very important that inflammation is contained, and chronic inflammation is fought with medicines, supplements, foods or through a combination of all in order to reduce or prevent it from happening.

Curcumin, the main active ingredient in turmeric, has high anti-inflammatory properties and some studies have shown that it can be as good as some anti-inflammatory drugs without any side effects.

Ginger has been used for centuries as an anti-inflammatory herb. Recent studies have shown that a steady intake of ginger for a period of more than a month helped reduce inflammation in the colon. By reducing inflammation, the risk of colon cancer is also reduced. Another study has shown promise in reducing inflammation associated with osteoarthritis.

Allicin, the sulfur compound in garlic, has high anti-inflammatory properties that stimulate the body's defenses and disease-fighting capabilities and helps fight inflammation effectively.

By fighting inflammation that weakens the body's immune system and damages cells, these spices help improve the body's defenses against cancer and other major diseases.

IMMUNE SYSTEM AND INFECTIONS

Turmeric, ginger, and garlic, with their antibacterial and antimicrobial properties, all have the capability to fight infections and boost the immune system. A body that is weak in its defenses against foreign invaders into the body is always at high risk for cancer and many other diseases. In addition, ginger has excellent capabilities to help maintain a healthy digestive system and stomach. A significant part of the body's immunity results from a healthy gut, and thus maintaining a healthy digestive system enhances the body's overall immunity and helps reduce the risk of not only cancer but many other diseases.

Cancer Prevention

The next chapter discusses other benefits of turmeric, ginger, and garlic. Many of these benefits contribute to overall health which in turn helps reduce cancer risk.

Chapter 6. Other Health Benefits of Turmeric, Ginger & Garlic

Turmeric has several uses and benefits. Its uses vary from cooking to food preservation to beauty enhancements and wound healing. Turmeric may be one of the most effective herbal nutritional supplements in existence. When consumed as a supplement or through food as part of cooking or preparation, it provides several additional health benefits.

The ginger root, when consumed regularly helps improve the digestive system. Ginger is known to reduce the feeling of nausea, and also improve your body's immune system to help fight common ailments such as flu, common cold, fever, and more.

Garlic was used by ancient civilizations primarily as an herb that provided some medicinal and health benefits. Later, garlic found its way into cooking for its unique taste and flavor. Today garlic is used in many cuisines starting from Chinese to Indian curries to Italian pizzas and pasta. Garlic is often an essential ingredient in meat preparation in India. While ancient civilizations used garlic for many ailments, there are a number of benefits that are identified as part of modern herbal medicine. Some of these benefits have been studied but a lot of work needs to be done to utilize these properties in mainstream treatments.

ARTHRITIS

Arthritis is a common health condition characterized by inflammation of joints. Due to its powerful anti-inflammatory characteristics, it is not surprising that turmeric can be effective in treating various kinds of arthritis. Several studies have been conducted that have shown that turmeric is effective in reducing pain, joint inflammation, and discomfort in rheumatoid arthritis (RA) which is one of the most common autoimmune diseases. Curcumin in turmeric is known to block inflammatory cytokines and enzymes. Some recent studies have shown that turmeric is effective in preventing RA as well as providing long term benefits, and some anecdotal reports have indicated that curcumin extract is effective in dogs with arthritis.

NEURO-PROTECTIVE

There have been multiple studies on the potential of turmeric for treating Alzheimer's and Parkinson's diseases. Much of this research is focused on antioxidant, anti-inflammatory, and anti-amyloid properties.

Though it has not been conclusively proven, there is some anecdotal evidence that turmeric could prevent the formation or even break up the amyloid-beta plaques considered to be associated with Alzheimer's disease.

Another compound in turmeric called turmerone has been shown in some studies to help create new brain cells by stimulating stem cells. This could help with arresting neurodegenerative conditions and help reduce the mental decline as people age.

Inflammation and oxidative damage to brain cells is considered the key contributing factors to the accelerated aging process. By consuming anti-oxidant and anti-inflammatory foods, one can reduce the effect of aging on the brain.

Ginger has antioxidant and anti-inflammatory properties that can help with slowing down the age-related decline in brain function such as Alzheimer's disease.

Garlic is a super brain food that has great properties to help slow down aging and age-related disorders. Garlic's antioxidant and anti-inflammatory properties combined with effects in reducing cholesterol and blood pressure may help slow down brain diseases like Alzheimer's and dementia.

CHOLESTEROL

Research has shown that feeding lab animals with turmeric extract resulted in reducing bad cholesterol and increasing good cholesterol, thereby reducing total cholesterol levels. In most studies, the improvements were in the 25-50% range. Curcumin's antioxidant property helps prevent oxidation of cholesterol, helps increase the metabolism of cholesterol, and reduces build-up.

Studies have shown that a daily intake of ginger helps reduce LDL cholesterol (bad cholesterol). The studies were conducted on humans as well as animals. As a result, the daily use of ginger may help maintain not only a healthy gut but a healthy heart as well.

Cancer Prevention

Garlic is believed to reduce both LDL (bad) cholesterol and total cholesterol. A number of research studies in humans and animals have found that the sulfur compounds in garlic help reduce LDL cholesterol and total cholesterol while they have no impact on HDL (good) cholesterol levels.

PAIN

With its anti-inflammatory and antioxidant properties, it is no wonder that turmeric is an effective remedy for pain, especially joint pains as a result of inflammation or arthritis. Some studies in rats have shown that turmeric naturally activated the body's inherent pain-relieving mechanisms.

Ginger is considered to help with pain – especially exercise-induced muscle pain. Drinking some ginger juice/drink after exercise regularly may be useful to relieve muscle pain. In addition, ginger has been studied for its effectiveness for menstrual pain and cramps and has been found as effective as some of the pain medications.

IMPROVED CIRCULATION

Studies have shown that curcumin has properties that help in unclogging your arteries and improving blood circulation. Turmeric could be considered a natural alternative to some of the common medications that help prevent blood clotting. A recent study in Japan showed that curcumin improved blood circulation in a trial group the same as a group that did regular exercise.

ANTI-DEPRESSANT

Studies conducted in India comparing curcumin and Prozac have shown that it has the same effect as Prozac in managing depression and could be considered as an effective and safe alternative for cases of mild depression.

GASTRO-INTESTINAL BENEFITS

Studies have shown several benefits for turmeric in gastrointestinal problems. Turmeric stimulates the gallbladder to produce more bile, which helps in digestion and promotes intestinal flora. Due to its anti-inflammatory properties, several inflammatory bowel diseases such as Chron's and Ulcerative Colitis could benefit from turmeric intake. The usage of turmeric helps to heal the digestive system and supports the growth of good bacteria.

SKIN AND HAIR

Turmeric is both a powerful antioxidant and an anti-inflammatory agent, but it also has anti-bacterial and anti-microbial properties. Therefore, it is no surprise that turmeric can do wonders for your skin. Turmeric is known to help in many problems associated with skin conditions and wound healing and it has also been used in the east (especially in India) as part of beauty-enhancing skin treatments.

Pastes containing turmeric are used for treating acne, eczema, and rosacea. By applying a turmeric facial mask or paste, one can reduce skin inflammation and redness associated with eczema or rosacea skin conditions.

In some Middle Eastern countries, garlic is used as a remedy for hair loss. Fresh garlic juice or garlic oil in combination with essential oils may be applied to the scalp. There is some evidence to suggest that garlic treatment may arrest hair loss or in some cases even promote hair growth.

Indigestion

Ginger has been used in traditional medicine as a digestive aid for thousands of years. In the East, ginger is an essential ingredient in meat cooking not only to add flavor to the food but also to help in digestion as well. Chewing on fresh ginger or drinking ginger juice/drink can help cure minor tummy aches (due to indigestion) and help with bloating and constipation.

Ginger relieves and relaxes gastrointestinal muscles that help reduce stomach irritation. It also helps in bile production and movement of food through the gastrointestinal tract thereby helping proper metabolism and food absorption in the body.

Nausea and Morning Sickness

Ginger has been used as a home remedy for different forms of nausea from morning sickness and motion sickness to even nausea due to chemotherapy.

Ginger has been used for motion sickness (seasickness primarily) for centuries. Recent studies have shown that ginger is effective in preventing both morning sickness and pregnancy-related nausea.

Diabetes and Heart Health

Ginger is believed to have several properties that help in maintaining a healthy heart including blood thinning, stimulating circulation, reducing cholesterol levels, and preventing heart attacks and strokes.

A study conducted on gingerol's effect on blood sugar found that there were significant benefits to using ginger powder in lowering blood sugar levels in diabetic patients.

LOWER BLOOD PRESSURE

Elevated blood pressure or hypertension is one of the key contributors to heart diseases such as heart attacks and strokes.

A number of studies in humans have found that a daily intake of garlic has very beneficial effects in lowering hypertension. In some studies, these benefits were as good as prescription medications.

IMPROVED PHYSICAL PERFORMANCE

Egyptians, Greeks, and Romans used to feed garlic to their warriors as well as slaves in hopes of improving their performance in the war or their slave output. Ancient Greeks fed garlic to Olympic athletes believing that garlic improved their physical capabilities, helping them win competitions. Garlic could be considered one of the earliest performance-enhancing substances.

COLD AND FLU

Allicin, the sulfur compound found in garlic has anti-microbial, anti-fungal, and anti-virus capabilities. As a result, garlic can help fight a number of common ailments that rise out of bacteria, fungal or viral infections.

In several studies conducted on the effectiveness of garlic, regular consumption of garlic was found to be effective in 1) preventing cold and flu and 2) speedy recovery in cases where the subjects of the study did catch a cold.

Bone Health

Garlic contains a number of minerals and vitamins that are considered the foundation for bone health such as zinc, manganese, Vitamin-B6, and Vitamin-C. In addition, regular use of garlic can increase estrogen in females helping to fight bone loss and osteoarthritis.

Antibacterial and Anti-parasitic

Allicin, the active ingredient in garlic, is an extremely anti-bacterial and antiparasitic compound. Allicin protects the garlic plant from fungus, bacteria, and parasites while growing in the soil. This property of allicin is also effective in humans when consumed. There has been a lot of evidence of garlic helping to fight common infections such as cold, flu, ear infection, etc. This is one of the reasons garlic was used as a remedy for plague and smallpox during medieval times.

Removing Splinters

Crushed garlic taped to a splinter that is either too small or too deep to remove, such as thorns, overnight can do wonders in removing the irritating splinter. Garlic can also help remove cold sores and even warts.

Detox Agent

Garlic with its anti-fungal, anti-bacterial, and anti-parasitic properties is a very good detox agent for the body. In addition, allicin, the sulfur compound in garlic, can neutralize heavy metals, especially neutralizing lead toxicity in the body.

Chapter 7. Recipes with the Cancer Fighting Trio of Spices – Turmeric, Ginger & Garlic

General tips for using turmeric, ginger, and garlic

There are several ways to incorporate turmeric, ginger, and garlic into your diet – both individually and together.

- Add ½ -1 teaspoon of turmeric powder and a pinch of black pepper powder when sautéing onions, herbs, or vegetables.

- Sauté crushed garlic and ginger in oil first before sautéing veggies or meats.

- Add a small piece of ginger/ turmeric root or both to the blender while making a smoothie.

- Add turmeric powder while making marinades and sauces.

- Make your own curry powder – by mixing 1 part turmeric, 1 part chili powder, 1 part coriander powder and optional roasted and ground fenugreek, cumin and mustard seeds.

- Add ½-1 teaspoon turmeric powder and a pinch of black pepper powder while making your favorite soup.

- Pickle garlic in vinegar.

- Roast garlic and use it to top salads.

Cancer Prevention

- Use garlic oil.
- Add ginger powder while baking.
- Add ginger paste (or ginger-garlic paste) to your marinades for grilling meat or fish.
- Add fresh ginger in making tea.
- Chew a piece of raw ginger (good for an upset stomach and nausea).
- Chew 1-2 garlic cloves raw every day.
- Add 1-2 cloves of garlic to the blender while making a smoothie.
- Make a paste of garlic and use it as part of a marinade for meats.

Drinks

Turmeric, ginger, and garlic may be used to make drinks such as tea, smoothies and others. There are several ways to make teas with ginger and turmeric. Fresh turmeric or ginger root may be added to smoothies along with other fruits or vegetables. While making smoothies, remember that adding a pinch of black pepper or fat such as coconut oil or flaxseed oil helps the absorption of curcumin, turmeric's active ingredient.

Basic Turmeric Tea

Ingredients:

- ½ - 2 teaspoon turmeric powder or ½ inch – 2 inch long fresh turmeric root grated (start with ½ teaspoon and increase the amount as you develop taste for turmeric)
- 1 tsp honey (or as much as desired to sweeten the tea to your taste)
- Pinch of freshly ground black pepper or pepper powder
- 1-2 cups of water

Method

1. Put the turmeric and ground pepper in a cup or pot, add one teaspoon of water, mix and make it into a paste.
2. Boil 1-2 cups of water and add to the turmeric paste. Mix it well.
3. Strain out the turmeric pieces, if any.
4. Let it cool for a couple of minutes and add honey. Enjoy warm.

Basic Ginger Tea

Ingredients:

- ½-2 inch fresh ginger grated
- 1 tsp honey (or as much to sweeten the tea to your taste)
- 1 tsp fresh lemon juice
- 1-2 cups of water

Method

1. Add grated ginger to water and boil it for a couple of minutes.
2. Let it cool for a couple of minutes.
3. Filter ginger slices; add honey and lemon juice; stir and enjoy lukewarm.

Basic Mushroom Tea

Ingredients:

- 1 chaga mushroom tea bag
- 1-2 cups of water

Method

1. Add the tea bag to the boiling water. Drink once a day

Notes:

1. Do not use if you are on blood-thinning or other medications. Consult a doctor
2. Chaga, Turkey Tail and Reishi mushroom powders, extracts and elixir are available through Amazon and other online stores
3. The same steps may be used in making dandelion tea which is considered good for cancer.

Cancer Prevention

BLACK TEA WITH GINGER AND CARDAMOM

Ingredients:

- ½-1 inch fresh ginger peeled and sliced/crushed
- 1 tsp honey (or as much as desired to sweeten the tea to your taste)
- 1-2 cups of water
- 1 black tea bag
- 2 cardamom pods
- ½ teaspoon lemon juice (optional)

Method

1. Add the ginger slices and optional cardamom to 1-2 cups of water and boil.
2. Add the black tea bag.
3. Let it cool for a couple of minutes.
4. Remove tea bag, filter ginger slices; add honey, and enjoy warm.

You can also try the same with the addition of an optional ½ teaspoon lemon juice.

Cancer Prevention

TURMERIC TEA WITH GINGER

Ingredients

- ½ - 2 teaspoon turmeric powder or ½ inch – 2 inch long fresh turmeric root grated
- ½ inch – 1 inch fresh ginger grated or thinly sliced
- 1 tsp honey (or as much to sweeten the tea to your taste)
- Pinch of freshly ground black pepper or pepper powder
- 1-2 cups of water

Method

1. Put the turmeric, ground pepper, and ginger in a cup or pot and add one spoon of water, mix and make it into a paste.
2. Boil 1-2 cups of water and add to the turmeric and ginger paste. Mix it well.
3. Strain out the ginger/turmeric pieces. Let it cool for a couple of minutes, add honey, and enjoy warm.

Cancer Prevention

HOT TURMERIC MILK

Basic Ingredients

- ½ - 2 teaspoon turmeric powder or ½ inch – 2 inch long fresh turmeric root grated (start with ½ teaspoon and increase the amount as you develop taste for turmeric)
- ½ inch – 1 inch fresh ginger grated or thinly sliced
- 1 tsp honey (or as much as desired to sweeten the tea to your taste)
- 1 pinch of freshly ground black pepper or pepper powder
- 1-2 cups of milk of your choice (regular, coconut or almond)

Optional Ingredients:

- 1 pinch of ground cloves
- ¼ teaspoon ground cardamom

Method

1. Mix turmeric, cardamom, black pepper, and cloves in a bowl.
2. Boil 1-2 cups of milk, add the turmeric mixture, and mix well. Careful not to boil over.
3. Strain out any lumps if need be. Let it cool for a couple of minutes and enjoy as it is or add honey/sugar and enjoy warm.

Green Tea with Turmeric & Ginger

Ingredients

- ½ - 2 teaspoon turmeric powder or ½ inch – 2 inches long fresh turmeric root
- ½ inch – 1 inch fresh ginger grated or thinly sliced
- 1 tsp honey (or as much as desired to sweeten the tea to your taste)
- 1 pinch of freshly ground black pepper or pepper powder
- 1-2 cups of green tea.

Method

1. Process all the ingredients in a blender until smooth.
2. Add the hot green tea, mix well.
3. Filter if needed. Add honey and enjoy it.

Recipe Note:

If using fresh turmeric root, either grind it as part of the rest of the ingredients or boil the root in 1-2 cups of water and green tea for 5 minutes on low heat. Then add pepper and honey once it cools down.

Masala Chai (Spiced Tea)

There are several ways to make masala chai. When I make it, I only use ginger and cardamom. The other ingredients to add based on one's taste are cinnamon, cloves, and pepper and fennel seeds.

Basic Ingredients

- ½ inch – 1 inch fresh peeled ginger grated, or crushed
- 4-6 cardamoms, crushed
- 1 inch long cinnamon stick or ¼ tsp cinnamon powder
- 2-4 tsp brown sugar (optional)
- ½ cup 2% milk
- 3 cups of water
- 2-4 tsp black tea or 2-3 tea bags

Optional Ingredients

- 2-4 cloves
- ¼ tsp pepper powder or about 4 peppercorns
- ¼ teaspoon fennel seeds

Method

1. Grind or crush cardamom, cinnamon, cloves, fennel seeds, and pepper in a spice grinder or mortar.
2. In a pan, add the ground mix and ginger and pour in 3 cups of water. Mix it well and bring it to a boil.
3. Reduce heat and let it simmer for a minute or two.
4. Now add the tea, mix, and let it boil for one minute on low heat.

5. Add milk and sugar and mix well. Strain out all the ingredients and enjoy.

If you have not tried masala chai before, I suggest you start with ginger and cardamom and then introduce other items before settling on the ingredient you like best.

Ginger and lemon tea

Ingredients

- ½ inch – 1 inch fresh ginger grated or crushed
- ½ tsp lemon juice
- 1 tsp honey
- 2 cups of water

Method

1. Boil 2 cups of water in a saucepan.
2. Add ginger and let it boil for 2-3 minutes.
3. Remove from heat and add lemon. Add honey and enjoy lukewarm

Note: This drink is good for nausea. Drink as often as needed.

GINGER ALE

Ingredients

- 1 cup ginger, peeled and sliced or crushed
- 2-3 cups of water
- ½ -1 cup brown sugar
- 1 spoon freshly squeezed lemon juice

Method

1. Add ginger to boiling water and simmer it for 10-15 minutes. Stir well.
2. Add sugar and let it fully dissolve.
3. Turn off the heat and let it sit until warm.
4. Strain the ginger pieces. Add lemon juice and stir. Pour the contents into a glass jar and refrigerate it.

The mixture may be used as-is (one tablespoon at a time) for nausea and indigestion or heartburn. You can also add 4-5 teaspoons of this mixture into a glass of club soda and drink.

TROPICAL SMOOTHIE

Ingredients

- ½ - 2 teaspoon turmeric powder or ½ inch – 2 inches long fresh turmeric root, cleaned and sliced (start with ½ teaspoon and increase the amount as you develop a taste for turmeric)
- ½ inch – 1 inch fresh ginger grated or thinly sliced
- 1 tsp honey (optional to taste)
- 1 pinch of freshly ground black pepper or pepper powder
- 1 banana
- 1 cup pineapple, mango or papaya
- 1 cup of milk or ½ cup plain yogurt
- ½ cup ice

Method

Process all the ingredients in a blender until smooth.

Green Smoothie with Garlic, Ginger, and Turmeric

Basic Ingredients

- ½ - 2 teaspoon turmeric powder or ½ inch – 2 inches long fresh turmeric root, cleaned and sliced
- ½ inch – 1 inch fresh ginger grated or thinly sliced
- 1-2 cloves garlic
- 1 pinch of freshly ground black pepper or pepper powder
- 1 cup kale, chopped
- 1 cup spinach
- 1-2 kiwis peeled
- ½ cup blueberries
- 1-2 cups filtered water (coconut water may be used as well)
- ½ cup ice

Optional Ingredients

- ½ cup cucumber, sliced
- ¼ avocado
- 1 tsp honey (or to taste)
- 3-4 mint leaves

Method

Process all the ingredients in a blender until smooth. Blueberries may be substituted with blackberries depending on your liking. Serves 3-4. By mixing and matching the "green" ingredients, you may try a couple of different green smoothies.

Cancer Prevention

GOLDEN YELLOW SMOOTHIE

Ingredients

- ½ - 2 teaspoon turmeric powder or ½ inch – 2 inches long fresh turmeric root, cleaned and sliced
- ½ inch – 1 inch fresh ginger grated or thinly sliced
- 1 tsp honey (optional to taste)
- 1 tsp coconut oil or butter
- 1 carrot washed and cut into pieces
- 1 mango peeled and sliced
- 1 cup orange or mango juice
- ½ cup ice

Method

Process all the ingredients in a blender until smooth.

VERY BERRY SMOOTHIE

Ingredients

- ½ inch – 1 inch fresh ginger, grated or thinly sliced
- 1 tsp honey (optional to taste)
- ½ cup blueberries
- ½ cup blackberries
- ½ cup raspberries
- ½ cup strawberries
- 1 cup 2% milk or lowfat yogurt
- ½ cup ice

Method

Process all the ingredients in a blender until smooth.

GARLIC DRINK WITH APPLE CIDER VINEGAR, LIME, AND HONEY

Ingredients:

- 10-12 cloves of garlic (about 1 full garlic bulb), peeled
- 1 lemon
- 2 cups of water
- ¼ cup raw unfiltered apple cider vinegar
- 2-4 tsp honey or to taste

Method

1. Squeeze the cloves completely to extract juice from garlic. You should get about 2 tsp from 1 bulb of garlic. Keep separate.
2. Juice lemon and keep separate.
3. In a pan heat the 2 cups of water to lukewarm.
4. Add vinegar, garlic, lemon juice, and honey. Mix well.

Consume ½ a cup 1-2 times a day and refrigerate any leftover to consume later.

This drink fights cold, flu, and other infections besides providing all of the other health benefits described.

Note: Instead of throwing away the residue from making garlic juice, it may be used when sautéing vegetables or cooking other food as described later.

GARLIC TEA WITH GINGER AND LEMON

Ingredients

- 1-2 cloves of garlic crushed
- ½ inch fresh ginger grated or thinly sliced

- 1 tsp honey (or as much as desired to sweeten the tea to your taste)
- 1 tsp lemon juice
- 2 cups of water
- pinch of black pepper powder (optional)

Method

1. Boil 2 cups of water, add crushed garlic and ginger and let it boil for 1 minute.
2. Add optional pepper.
3. Switch off the heat and let it sit for 20 minutes.
4. Strain out the ginger/garlic pieces. Let it cool for a couple of minutes
5. Add honey and lemon juice and enjoy warm.

This drink is good for digestion, fighting cold/flu, clearing nasal congestion, sore throat, etc.

Note: Optionally 2 tsp apple cider vinegar also may be added to the boiled water along with the rest of the ingredients.

RED WINE AND GARLIC

Ingredients

- 1 bulb of garlic (about 10-12 cloves), peeled and chopped
- ½ liter red wine

Method

1. Pour the wine into a glass bottle, add the chopped garlic and mix well.
2. Close the glass bottle tightly and keep it exposed to sunlight for 2 weeks (near a window possibly)
3. Shake the jar a couple of times a day to make sure the contents are mixed well.
4. After letting the mixture sit for about 2 weeks, filter the garlic out, store the wine in a glass bottle and refrigerate.

The drink may be consumed directly 1-2 teaspoons two times a day. It can also be used as a salad dressing or for cooking.

Cancer Prevention

GARLIC AND LEMON DRINK

Ingredients

- 3 full garlic bulbs (about 100gm) cloves, peeled and chopped.
- 4 lemons washed and chopped
- 4-5 tsp honey (optional)
- 3-4 cups of water

Method

1. Add garlic and lemons to boiling water and keep it boiling on low heat for 15 minutes.
2. Switch off the heat and let it cool down. Add honey and refrigerate in a glass jar.

Drink 3 tablespoons daily until the drink is finished. Take a pause 2-3 weeks before making and consuming this again.

Note:

This is an adapted recipe from www.healthyfoodteam.com. This is a natural remedy against cancer-causing bad cells, helping to improve cholesterol and clearing clogged arteries.

YOGURT WITH TURMERIC, GINGER, AND GARLIC OR YOGURT CURRY

This is a popular curry in Indian cooking and has several different variations. The simplest version of the recipe is below.

Basic Ingredients

- 1 teaspoon turmeric powder
- ½ inch – 1 inch fresh ginger, grated or thinly sliced
- 2-3 cloves of garlic chopped
- 1 pinch of black pepper powder
- 2 cups of yogurt whisked
- 1 medium onion finely chopped
- 2 tsp coconut (or vegetable) oil
- Salt to taste

Optional Ingredients

- ¼ cup cilantro or curry leaves chopped
- 1 tsp mustard seeds
- 1 tsp cumin seeds
- 2 crushed red chilies

Method:

1. Heat oil in a medium non-stick pan, add optional mustard seeds, cumin, and red chilies and let it crackle
2. Add onions, ginger, garlic, and optional curry leaves or cilantro.
3. Stir until golden and add turmeric and black pepper, stir for one minute and then add the yogurt and mix well. Switch off the heat and enjoy it with rice.

Entrées and Other Dishes

Kale chips

Ingredients

- One bunch of red, green, or Lacinato kale
- 2 tsp olive oil or garlic oil
- a pinch of salt (optional)

Method

1. Preheat the oven to 350 degrees Fahrenheit (175 C).
2. Use a knife to remove the thick stem from the leaves (the thick stem may be reused in soups or chili instead of discarding) and then tear the leaves into small chip-sized pieces.
3. Put all the pieces in a mixing bowl and sprinkle with oil (olive or garlic oil) and optional salt (kale is a bit salty by itself so you can skip the salt depending on your taste) and mix well. Set it aside for 5 minutes before baking.
4. Bake for 10 minutes or until the kale pieces are crisp (be careful not to burn the chips).

Spinach/Red Chard Stir Fry

Basic Ingredients

- 4 cup spinach or red chard chopped
- ½ cup onions, chopped
- 4-5 cloves of garlic, crushed
- 1 tsp turmeric powder
- 2 tsp coconut oil (or vegetable oil)
- Salt to taste
- 1 cup grated coconut

Optional Ingredients

- 2-3 dry red chilies
- 1 spring curry leaves
- ½ tsp mustard seeds
- 1 tsp cumin seeds

Method

1. Heat oil in a non-stick pan. Add optional mustard and cumin seeds and let it splutter.
2. Add onions, garlic, optional curry leaves, and red chilies, sauté for a couple of minutes until onions become translucent.
3. Add turmeric powder and sauté for a couple of minutes more.
4. Now add the chopped spinach or red chard and mix well. Cover and cook for 5-7 minutes stirring occasionally to make sure no water remains.
5. Add grated coconut, and salt and mix well.
6. Cook on low flame for 5 more minutes stirring occasionally. Switch off the heat once spinach/chard is cooked and there is no water remains.

Salmon with Green Mango

Cancer Prevention

Basic Ingredients

- 2lbs. skinless salmon, cleaned and cut into 2 inch pieces
- 1-4 tsp chili powder, (depending on your tolerance level)
- 1 tsp turmeric powder
- 1 tsp coriander powder
- ¼ tsp fenugreek powder or ½ tsp fenugreek seeds
- ¼ tsp black pepper powder
- ½ tsp mustard seeds
- 1 medium onion, sliced
- 2 tsp ginger, grated
- 4-5 cloves garlic, crushed
- 2 cups green mango, cashed and cut into 1 inch pieces (with skin or skin removed depending on your preference)
- 1 to 1.5 cups water (or as required)
- salt to taste

Optional Ingredients

- 2 springs curry leaves
- 2-4 sliced green chilies or jalapeños, seeds removed

Method

1. Combine all the spice powders – chili, turmeric, coriander, fenugreek, and pepper powder - together in a bowl. Add 2 tsp or just enough water to make a thick paste and set aside.
2. Heat oil in a pan and splutter mustard seeds and fenugreek (if seeds are used instead of powder).

3. Add ginger, garlic, onion, and optional green chilies and curry leaves. Sauté until onion becomes translucent.
4. Add the masala paste and mix well on low flame (wet the masala to make sure it gets fried but not burnt).
5. After a few minutes (once masala gets fried), add about 2 cups of water, mix, and then add the cut mango pieces.
6. Cover it and bring it a boil on medium heat. Now add individual fish pieces into the pan.
7. Mix gently, making sure the fish pieces are not broken up and that all the pieces are coated with the gravy.
8. Cover the pan and cook it for about 20 minutes or until fish is done and the gravy is thick. Switch off the flame and keep it covered for 30 minutes for the fish to soak in the spices and mango flavor.

Serve with rice or bread.

Notes:

1. Paprika may be used instead of chili powder if you desire to make it less spicy.
2. Any other fish may be used instead of salmon.
3. Instead of mango, tamarind, or *Garcinia cambogia* (the scientific name for black tamarind available in Asian stores) may be used.
4. Green chilies or jalapeños add more heat to the fish curry. Use them depending on your taste.

Cancer Prevention

BROCCOLI STIR FRY

Basic Ingredients

- 2 lb. broccoli florets washed
- 2 tsp coconut oil (olive oil or vegetable oil can be used instead)
- 1 tsp turmeric powder
- 1 medium onion sliced
- ¼ tsp black pepper powder
- Salt to taste

Optional Ingredients

- 1 Jalapeño pepper sliced into thin pieces (seeds out)
- 1 tsp mustard seeds
- ½ cup fresh cilantro
- ½ cup fresh parsley
- ½ tsp fresh lemon juice

Method

1. Heat oil in a medium non-stick pan; crackle optional mustard seeds in oil.
2. Add onions and optional jalapeño peppers. Stir until golden.
3. Add turmeric and black pepper, stir for one minute, and then add broccoli florets and mix well until the broccoli is coated with the turmeric.
4. Cover the pan with a lid and cook for 5-10 minutes on low-medium heat, stirring occasionally. Once cooked,

switch off heat; add the optional cilantro and parsley. Add salt to taste. Add optional lemon juice.

Mix well and serve hot. Usually, there is no need to add water. At low heat, the moisture in broccoli will help it to cook well.

BELL PEPPER AND CHICKEN STIR FRY

Basic Ingredients

- 1 bell pepper washed and cut into thin slices
- 2 tsp coconut oil (olive oil or vegetable oil can be used instead)
- 1 lb. boneless chicken breast cut into thin strips
- 1 tsp turmeric powder
- 1 tsp black pepper powder
- 1 tsp coriander powder
- 1 medium onion sliced
- ½ inch fresh ginger root, thinly sliced
- salt to taste
- 1-2 medium tomatoes sliced
- 3 cloves of garlic crushed

Optional Ingredients

- 1 Jalapeño pepper sliced into thin pieces
- ¼ cup fresh cilantro chopped

Method

1. Sprinkle ½ teaspoons of turmeric powder, pepper powder, and salt on the washed and cut chicken, mix well and set aside for 10 minutes.
2. In a pan, heat oil and add onions, crushed garlic, ginger, and optional Jalapeno. Sauté till onions become translucent.

3. Add the rest of turmeric powder, coriander powder, and pepper powder and mix well.
4. Add tomato and mix.
5. Now add the bell pepper and chicken and mix well.
6. Cover and cook for 10 minutes on medium heat or until chicken and peppers are cooked. Stir occasionally.
7. Switch off the heat, add optional cilantro and add more salt if required depending on your taste.

Serve with rice or bread

Cancer Prevention

COCONUT CURRY CHICKEN

Basic Ingredients

- 1-1/2 pound chicken breast cut into small (1 inch) pieces
- 2-4 teaspoons of curry powder depending on your tolerance to the spice
- 1 tsp turmeric
- 1` medium onion chopped
- 2-3 tsp coconut oil (olive oil or vegetable oil can be used instead)
- ½ tsp black pepper powder
- 2 medium potatoes, peeled and cut into 1 inch cubes
- 3-4 cloves of garlic crushed
- ½ inch cube of ginger peeled and sliced
- 1 can (14 oz) of coconut milk
- ¼ cup fresh mint leaves or cilantro
- ¼ tsp salt (or to taste)
- ½ -1 can of chicken broth (depending on the amount of gravy desired)

Optional Ingredients

- 1 cup carrots, sliced
- 2 medium tomatoes, chopped

Method

1. Sprinkle 1 tsp curry powder, ½ tsp turmeric, and ¼ tsp salt on cut chicken. Mix well and keep it aside for 10 minutes.

Cancer Prevention

2. In a separate pan, heat oil and sauté onion, garlic, and ginger until onion becomes translucent.
3. Add remaining curry powder, turmeric, and pepper powder. Mix for 1-2 minutes.
4. Add chicken, potatoes, and optional tomatoes and carrots. Mix well 1-2 minutes until the chicken and potatoes are coated with the gravy.
5. Add chicken broth and bring it to a boil. Stir well.
6. Reduce heat to low medium, cover the pan and cook for 10-12 minutes or until chicken, potatoes and carrots are well mixed and chicken loses its pink color and potatoes and carrots are about half cooked.
7. Add coconut milk and cover. Simmer on low heat for another 20 minutes or until chicken, potatoes and carrots are cooked well and soft.
8. Add mint leaves/cilantro and stir. Add salt to taste.
9. Switch off the heat and keep it covered for 1-2 minutes before serving.

Serve with rice or bread.

Cancer Prevention

CAULIFLOWER AND POTATO

Basic Ingredients

- 2 medium potatoes, peeled and cut into 1 inch cubes
- ½ head of cauliflower washed and cut into small pieces (same size as the potatoes)
- 2 tsp coconut oil (olive oil or coconut oil can be used instead)
- ½ tsp black pepper powder
- 1 medium onion sliced
- 1 tsp turmeric powder
- 1-2 medium tomatoes, chopped
- ¼ tsp salt (or to taste)
- ¼ cup fresh cilantro chopped
- ½ cup vegetable broth

Optional Ingredients
- ½ tsp cumin seeds
- 1-2 jalapenos sliced (seed out/in)
- 2-3 cloves of garlic crushed
- ½ inch fresh ginger root, chopped
- ½-1 tsp curry powder

Method

1. Heat oil in a medium non-stick pan, and crackle optional cumin seeds in oil.
2. Add onion, and optional garlic, ginger, and jalapenos. Stir until onion becomes translucent.
3. Add turmeric, black pepper, and optional curry powder and stir for 1-2 minutes.
4. Add chopped tomatoes, potatoes and cauliflower, mix well and then add vegetable broth.

5. Bring to a boil stirring in between.
6. Cover and simmer for 10-15 minutes, or until the potatoes and cauliflower are cooked.
7. Switch off heat; add the cilantro and salt.

Mix well and serve hot as a side dish with rice or bread.

Note 1: There are many optional ingredients listed, one could use all of them or pick and choose based on your tastes.

Note 2: The jalapenos vary in their heat level. If you choose to use them, you can take the seeds out to reduce the heat. This note applies to all the recipes in this book.

Cancer Prevention

TOMATO RICE

This is a good way to color your rice and also include turmeric, ginger, and garlic as part of the diet.

Basic Ingredients

- 2 cup basmati rice, uncooked
- 1 tsp turmeric powder
- 2 tsp coconut oil (olive oil or vegetable oil can be used instead)
- 1 pinch black pepper powder
- 3 medium tomatoes, chopped
- 1 medium onion, chopped
- ¼ tsp salt (or to taste)
- ¼ cup fresh cilantro chopped

Optional Ingredients

- ½ tsp mustard seeds
- ½ tsp cumin seeds
- 1-2 jalapenos sliced
- 3 cloves of garlic, crushed
- ½ inch piece of ginger, thinly sliced

Method

1. Cook the rice in a rice cooker or on stovetop drain (if needed) and set aside.
2. In a medium pan (big enough to mix rice), heat oil, and crackle optional mustard and seeds
3. Add onions, and optional garlic, ginger, and jalapenos; sauté until onions are golden brown.

4. Add turmeric and pepper and mix. Now add the tomatoes; mix.
5. Cover and cook for 10 minutes on medium heat or until tomatoes are cooked well.
6. Add the cooked rice, mix it well, and add salt to taste.
7. Add chopped cilantro and serve.

BEEF/CHICKEN PEPPER FRY

Ingredients

- 2 lb. boneless chicken breast/beef cut into 1 inch cubes/strips
- 2 tsp coconut oil (olive oil or vegetable oil can be used instead)
- 1/2 tsp turmeric powder
- 1-2 tsp black pepper powder
- 2 tsp coriander powder
- 2 large onion, sliced
- 2 inches of ginger, thinly sliced
- ¼ tsp salt (or to taste)
- 2-3 medium tomato sliced
- 4-6 cloves of garlic crushed

Optional Ingredients

- 1 cup fresh cilantro, chopped
- 1 Jalapenos, sliced

Method

1. Heat oil in a medium non-stick pan; add onions, garlic, ginger, and optional Jalapeno. Stir until golden.

2. Add coriander powder, pepper powder and turmeric. Stir for 2-3 minutes.
3. Add tomato and mix well.
4. Add chicken and mix so that chicken is coated well with spices and onions.
5. Cover and simmer for 20-25 minutes or until the chicken is cooked stirring occasionally so the chicken or the gravy does not stick to the pan.
6. Garnish with cilantro.

Serve with rice or naan (Indian bread).

GRILLED CHICKEN

Tandoori chicken is an Indian dish that is marinated in yogurt and spices and cooked in a clay oven. It invariably uses a ginger-garlic paste as part of the marinade. Below is a variation of tandoori chicken that is cooked on a grill.

Ingredients

- 2-3 lbs. whole skinless chicken drumsticks or whole thighs or boneless chicken breast cut into pieces.
- 2-3 tsp ginger-garlic paste (see earlier instructions to make it or use store-bought)
- 1 cup low-fat yogurt
- 1 tsp chili powder
- ¼ tsp turmeric powder
- 3 teaspoon tandoori masala (see note below)
- 1 lemon juiced
- 1 cup fresh cilantro (to garnish)
- 2 lemons sliced (to garnish)

- 1 medium onion sliced into long pieces (optional)
- 1 teaspoon salt (or to taste)
- 1 teaspoon coconut oil (olive oil or vegetable oil can be used instead)

Method

The first step is to prepare the marinade.

Marinade method 1: Mix all the items for the marinade (yogurt, chili, turmeric, tandoori masala, lemon juice and ginger/garlic paste, salt) into a smooth thick marinade.

Marinade method 2: Heat oil and fry chili powder, tandoori masala and turmeric for 2 minutes. Switch off the heat and let it cool down. Once cooled, add this to the rest of the ingredients of the marinade and mix well as in the previous step.

1. Put the chicken in a large freezer /zip lock bag and add the marinade. You may want to use multiple freezer bags depending on the quantity but make sure to put sufficient marinade in each bag. Shake the bag carefully so that the chicken is well coated with the marinade. Refrigerate for a minimum of 2 hours but preferably 12 hours or overnight.
2. When ready to cook, preheat oven to 400 degrees. Take the chicken out of the zip lock bags and carefully place the chicken on a wire rack on the baking dish. The baking dish may be lined with aluminum foil to collect any juice coming out of the chicken. Bake for 25 minutes. Open the oven and apply some oil using a brush on the surface of chicken pieces and turn them

over. Bake for another 20 minutes or until cooked well and slightly charred. Take it from oven. Garnish with cilantro, lemon wedges and optional onion slices.

Instead of using the oven, the marinated chicken may be barbecued or grilled on an open grill.

Note: You can substitute garam masala for tandoori masala. Both of these spice mixes are available in any South Asian store or in the spice section in many grocery stores. You can also make the spice mix by combining the following: 1 tsp coriander powder, 1 tsp pepper powder, 1 tsp cinnamon powder, 1 tsp turmeric powder, ½ tsp cardamom powder (or seeds), 1 tsp chili powder, and ½ tsp nutmeg.

KALE AND CHICKEN FRY

This is something I tried recently and found good. The simplest way to make this is to make chicken with spices following any one of the recipes above, make kale chips, and just crumble the chips into the chicken and mix well.

Ingredients

- 2 lb. boneless chicken breast/beef cut into 1 inch cubes/strips
- 2 tsp coconut oil (olive oil or vegetable oil can be used instead)
- 1/2 tsp turmeric powder
- 1-2 tsp black pepper powder
- 2 tsp coriander powder
- 2 large onions, sliced
- 2 inch piece of ginger thinly sliced
- Salt to taste
- 2-3 medium tomatoes, sliced
- 4-6 cloves of garlic crushed
- Cilantro – 1 cup (optional)
- 2 cups of green or red kale washed and cut/torn into 1-2 inch pieces (to make kale chips)

Method

1. Heat oil in a medium non-stick pan; add onions, garlic, and ginger. Stir until golden.
2. Add coriander powder, pepper powder and turmeric, stir for one minute and then add tomatoes and mix well.
3. Add chicken mix so that chicken is coated well with spices and onion.

Cancer Prevention

4. Cover and simmer for 20-25 minutes or until the chicken is cooked stirring occasionally so the chicken or the gravy does not stick to the pan.
5. Meanwhile in parallel, spread the kale pieces on a cookie sheet and put in the oven at 350 degrees for 10 minutes or until the kale becomes chips and can easily crumble.
6. Once the chicken is cooked, take the kale chips and crumble using your hand; spread it on top of chicken fry.
7. Mix well and cover it for 1 minute. Garnish with cilantro.

Serve with rice or naan (Indian bread).

CHAPTER 8. TIPS FOR BUYING & USING TURMERIC, GINGER & GARLIC

BUYING

Turmeric and ginger are available to buy in both fresh and dried root form as well as in powder form. Ginger can be found in most grocery stores while turmeric root is only available in specialty stores. While ginger is used mostly in fresh root form, turmeric is mostly used in the powder form and is available in Asian grocery stores or online.

Fresh garlic is available in most grocery stores. Garlic and ginger pastes or garlic-ginger pastes may be purchased from Asian stores.

Nutritional and supplement stores carry a wide variety of extracts of these three spices. All these extracts (turmeric, ginger, and garlic) are pretty popular as nutritional supplements.

COOKING

Turmeric, ginger, and garlic have been used in cooking for thousands of years. In South Asian cooking, all three of these spices are used together and with other spices such as chilies, cumin, and coriander to enhance the flavor, aroma, and color of the food to make it more appetizing as well as healthful. However, with the many health benefits of these spices, it is clear that a conscious, well thought out regimen of incorporating them makes the most sense.

As the studies have shown, curcumin, the active ingredient in turmeric, is not easily absorbed by the human body. Black pepper and fatty oils help increase the absorption very significantly. The simplest way to include turmeric in cooking is to sprinkle a mixture of turmeric powder and black pepper powder on the meat before grilling, searing, or pan-frying. Not only is this healthful and provides numerous benefits, but it also adds color to your food and makes it appealing. Another easy way is to add some turmeric and black pepper powder to your choice of marinade along with some ginger-garlic paste. Pieces of turmeric, ginger, and garlic may be added to soups or added while making smoothies/tea.

Garlic and ginger may be used together as a paste for marinades. Ginger teas provide relief to stomach ailments, nausea, the common cold, and sore throat.

Raw turmeric Vs. turmeric powder

While turmeric powder is convenient, raw turmeric is certainly more highly recommended than turmeric powder due to several reasons. Raw turmeric has better absorption, is pure (no additives and no loss of curcumin) and is easier to put into smoothies. Lastly, raw turmeric may be grown in your own backyard.

Ginger and garlic powders

While fresh ginger and garlic are always preferable and easier to buy, its powdered form is also easily available and offers more shelf life, so it is a worthy alternative to fresh ginger and garlic. The ginger powder may be added to tea, smoothies, or as part of a spice blend in cooking. Garlic powder may be added to vegetables while sautéing. Both garlic and ginger are perennials and may be grown in your own backyard.

GINGER PASTE

Ginger paste is often used as an alternative to fresh ginger and also as part of a marinade for grilling or baking meat. Ginger may be combined with garlic to make ginger garlic paste and stored for several days for use in cooking or marinating meat.

GARLIC PASTE

Garlic paste is often used as an alternative to fresh garlic in cooking and as part of a marinade for grilling or baking meat. Garlic may be combined with ginger to make ginger garlic paste and refrigerated for several days for use in cooking or marinating meat.

GINGER, GARLIC AND TURMERIC PASTE

Ginger and garlic paste are used often as part of a marinade in South Asian cooking. Almost all meat recipes use ginger and garlic as ingredients.

The steps below are for making a paste that contains not only ginger and garlic but turmeric as well. This is a powerful combination of ingredients that will not only make your meat tasty but also provide excellent health benefits as well.

Ingredients

- 1 cup ginger, washed, peeled, and cut into small pieces
- 1 cup garlic, peeled
- ¼ cup turmeric root, washed, peeled, and cut
- ½ -1 tsp salt
- 1 tsp vegetable oil

Method:

1. Make sure the ginger and turmeric are dried enough to remove any water from washing.
2. Add all ingredients into a blender and grind into a smooth paste.
3. Store the contents in a glass jar and use within 3-4 days or a week.

The paste may be used as part of any marinade for meat before grilling or baking in an oven or even cooking in a pan.

Garlic Oil

Garlic oil is available to purchase from many of the grocery stores or online retailers. A simple way to make garlic oil is by heating peeled and chopped garlic in an oil of your choice and frying them until they become opaque in color. Let it sit until cooled down to room temperature and filter out the garlic. The oil may be bottled and used for salads topical uses and for sautéing.

Dosage

Turmeric:

Most of the studies of curcumin have used a dosage of 600mg to 1200mg curcumin extract a day. Given that turmeric only contains 3% curcumin by weight, to achieve the suggested dosage levels using the turmeric spice in your foods alone is pretty difficult. So, a combination of food and supplements may be the optimal way to intake curcumin and exploit the many benefits.

Garlic:

Most of the studies of garlic have used a dosage of 1000mg to 2000mg garlic supplements a day. For children and pregnant women, the dosage is much lower. 2-5 grams of fresh raw garlic a day is considered a typical dosage. This translates into ½ to 1½ cloves a day. As always, discuss with your primary care provider before taking any supplements.

Ginger:

Studies using ginger have used a dosage of 1000mg to 3000mg per day. A combination of ginger, garlic, and turmeric is considered most effective, as it has been used in Asian cooking.

SUPPLEMENTS

Turmeric, ginger, and garlic extracts are available to buy from many online stores such as Amazon and other specialty health and nutritional stores. These capsules vary in dosage depending on the vendor and the ingredient (turmeric, garlic or ginger). Most of the dosages are usually 500mg – 1500mg extract. Several of these online stores have large testimonials on their effectiveness.

CHAPTER 9. SUMMARY

I hope this book provides you with some understanding of the cancer-causing factors to avoid as well as insight into the various cancer fighting foods. The use of spices and herbs, with their medicinal properties, help transform any meal into a healthful and disease fighting meal. While the book lists a number of external factors, the focus of this book remains on what you put into your body and how one can remove unhealthy eating habits. Here is my list of top 10 things to prevent cancer.

1. Be aware and conscious about what you eat or drink

- Eat more colorful vegetables and fruits
- Limit/avoid processed foods
- Limit/avoid sodas of any kind
- Eat more vegan and organic protein
- Limit sugar intake
- Limit alcohol
- Limit salt. Be aware many off the shelf and processed foods have too much sodium.
- Eat freshly prepared foods whenever possible. Cook at home more often. It makes not only short term and long-term economic sense but is healthful as well.

- Use spices and herbs – especially turmeric, garlic, and ginger (and others such as cinnamon, chili powder, etc.) in the preparation of food.

- Avoid food preservatives

2. Be physically active

- Be aware of how much time you exercise, and how much time you sit on the sofa or sit at the workplace

- Exercise at least 30 minutes a day. Pick up a physical activity that you enjoy. Enlist other people so you can exercise in groups or teams where you can feed off each other and maintain the motivation.

- Hit the gym or pick up running, walking or a team game such as tennis, volleyball, basketball, etc.

- Find out if Yoga or Tai chi is good for you.

- Reduce sitting and watching TV

3. Maintain closer to an ideal body weight

- Be aware of the ideal body weight for your height/weight/age/gender

- If it is above the ideal weight, take steps to reduce it. Even a 10-15% reduction in weight can help reduce cancer risk significantly.

Cancer Prevention

4. Be aware of the environmental factors

- Is your workplace safe and healthy?

- Are you exposed to harmful chemicals at work or at home?

- Limit the use of non-organic, unsafe cleaning products, and laundry detergents (avoid dry cleaning) in and around your home.

- Reduce the use of pesticides or use a safer variety

- Are there radiation sources around you? High tension transmission lines, excessive use of cell phones without a hands-free device, etc.

- Avoid exposure to smoke and other fumes

- Check your home for radon. Radon exposure is the number one cause of lung cancer among no-smokers in the US.

5. Avoid smoking

- Smoking and exposure to smoke are some of the easier cancer prevention things one can do. Research has shown without a doubt that smoking can cause lung cancer and other forms of pulmonary cancers.

6. Be aware of tanning solutions including sun exposure

- Sun exposure is the leading cause of skin cancer. Use an SPF 30 or higher sunblock solution. Apply liberally and as often as needed before going out into the sunshine. Avoid breathing sunblock sprays

| Cancer Prevention

- Avoid suntan salons whenever possible.

- Avoid excess UV rays natural (sun) or artificial (sun tanning salons). These are not good for your skin.

7. Be aware of your family's medical history

- While your DNA/genetics is something one cannot change, being aware of family history helps one to take preventive and cautionary steps that can certainly either completely prevent or reduce the risk of getting cancer

- Research your family history and understand what kind of cancer risk you are exposed to. You can take specific actions as well as share it with your doctor who can help devise a strategy against cancer.

8. Practice safe sex

- Human papillomavirus or HPV is the leading cause of cervical cancer. HPV virus often transmitted sexually (STD) and is responsible for a number of cancers.

9. Strengthen your gut or digestive system

- Your gut is the center of the body's immune system. Maintaining a strong and healthy digestive system is as important to preventing many diseases as other factors are.

- Eat pro-biotic foods – yogurt, kefir, kimchi, etc. This help increases the good bacteria in your gut

- Use spices such as ginger, turmeric, and garlic which are especially known to improve digestive health.

- Consider cancer fighting mushrooms and various teas

- Limit the use of antibiotics and use them only to cure bacterial infections. Antibiotics won't cure a common cold and flu as they are caused by viruses. Antibiotics kill the friendly bacteria in your stomach and as a result, weaken your immune system

- Fight common ailments such as cold, flu, cough, etc. with food and other remedies (for example ginger/turmeric/garlic teas and drinks described in this book) rather than antibiotics.

10. Refer back to the top 3 above!

- Again, the top three cancer prevention techniques are diet, exercise, and maintaining a healthy body. I cannot overemphasize this. One has complete control over these three while has no control or limited control over many others such as genetics and environmental factors.

So, if you can do one thing only that should be fixing what you put into your body. If you can combine diet with exercise you are on a path to a very healthy and hopefully cancer-free life.

I wish you all the best in your journey towards a cancer-free future!

Cancer Prevention

DISCLAIMER

This book details the author's personal experiences in using Indian spices and information contained in the public domain as well as the author's opinion. The author is not licensed as a doctor, nutritionist, or chef. The author is providing this book and its contents on an "as is" basis and makes no representations or warranties of any kind with respect to this book or its contents. The author disclaims all such representations and warranties, including for example warranties of merchantability and educational or medical advice for a particular purpose. In addition, the author does not represent or warrant that the information accessible via this book is accurate, complete, or current. The statements made about products and services have not been evaluated by the US FDA or any equivalent organization in other countries.

The author will not be liable for damages arising out of or in connection with the use of this book or the information contained within. This is a comprehensive limitation of liability that applies to all damages of any kind, including (without limitation) compensatory; direct, indirect or consequential damages; loss of data, income or profit; loss of or damage to property and claims of third parties. It is understood that this book is not intended as a substitute for consultation with a licensed medical or a culinary professional. Before starting any lifestyle changes, it is recommended that you consult a licensed professional to ensure that you are doing what's best for your situation. The use of this book implies your acceptance of this disclaimer.

Thank You

If you enjoyed this book or found it useful, I would greatly appreciate if you could post a short review on Amazon. I read all the reviews and your feedback will help me to make this book even better. For your convenience, please click the following link to take you directly to Amazon where you can post the review.

https://www.amazon.com/dp/B074N6Q8DT

Appendix I. Sources & References

This book was written based on the author's personal experience with the spice as well as information from a wide range of sources. Some of the key sources are outlined below, in case; the reader would like to read more details about cancer and its prevention.

Cancer

Perspectives on cancer prevention with natural compounds

http://cancerpreventionresearch.aacrjournals.org/content/6/5/387

The Amazing Cancer-Fighting Benefits of Curcumin

https://thetruthaboutcancer.com/cancer-fighting-benefits-of-curcumin/

http://www.riseearth.com/2016/06/the-amazing-cancer-fighting-benefits-of.html

Ginger is Stronger than Chemotherapy for Cancer

https://foodrevolution.org/blog/ginger-cancer-treatment/

Benefits of whole ginger extract in prostate cancer

https://www.ncbi.nlm.nih.gov/pubmed/21849094

Ginger inhibits cell growth and modulates angiogenic factors in ovarian cancer cells

https://www.ncbi.nlm.nih.gov/pubmed/18096028

Six foods that fight cancer:

http://www.foxnews.com/story/2006/04/27/six-foods-that-fight-cancer.html

The Amazing and Mighty Ginger

https://www.ncbi.nlm.nih.gov/books/NBK92775/

Phase II study of the Effects of Ginger Root Extract on Eicosanoids in Colon Mucosa in People at Normal Risk for Colorectal Cancer

https://www.ncbi.nlm.nih.gov/pmc/articles/PMC3208778/

Colon cancer: Symptoms, causes, and treatment

http://www.medicalnewstoday.com/articles/150496.php

Garlic and onions: Their cancer prevention properties

https://www.ncbi.nlm.nih.gov/pmc/articles/PMC4366009/

| Cancer Prevention

Garlic, onion and cereal fibre as protective factors for breast cancer: a French case-control study

https://www.ncbi.nlm.nih.gov/pubmed/9928867

Garlic and Organosulfer Compounds – Oregon State University

http://lpi.oregonstate.edu/mic/food-beverages/garlic#biological-activities-cancer-prevention

Can turmeric beat cancer – Cancer research UK

http://www.cancerresearchuk.org/about-cancer/cancers-in-general/cancer-questions/can-turmeric-prevent-bowel-cancer

Specific inhibition of cyclooxygenase-2 (COX-2) expression by dietary curcumin in HT-29 human colon cancer cells

http://www.cancerletters.info/article/S0304-3835(01)00655-3/fulltext?cc=y=

HYPERTENSION

Garlic supplementation prevents oxidative DNA damage in essential hypertension.

https://www.ncbi.nlm.nih.gov/pubmed/16335787

Aged garlic extract lowers blood pressure in patients with treated but uncontrolled hypertension: a randomized controlled trial.

https://www.ncbi.nlm.nih.gov/pubmed/20594781

Effects of *Allium sativum* (garlic) on systolic and diastolic blood pressure in patients with essential hypertension.

https://www.ncbi.nlm.nih.gov/pubmed/24035939

CHOLESTEROL & BLOOD PRESSURE

Lipid-lowering effects of time-released garlic powder tablets in double-blinded placebo-controlled randomized study.

https://www.ncbi.nlm.nih.gov/pubmed/19060427

Garlic for treating hypercholesterolemia. A meta-analysis of randomized clinical trials.

https://www.ncbi.nlm.nih.gov/pubmed/10975959

Investigation of the effect of ginger on the lipid levels. A double blind controlled clinical trial.

https://www.ncbi.nlm.nih.gov/pubmed/18813412

| Cancer Prevention

Antihyperlipidemic effects of ginger extracts in alloxan-induced diabetes and propylthiouracil-induced hypothyroidism in (rats).

https://www.ncbi.nlm.nih.gov/pubmed/23901210

Turmeric's Effects on High Blood Pressure and Cholesterol

http://www.turmeric.com/cardiovascular/turmerics-effects-on-high-blood-pressure-and-cholesterol

8 Proven Benefits of Turmeric for High Cholesterol

http://www.turmericforhealth.com/turmeric-benefits/turmeric-benefits-for-cholesterol

COLD & FLU

Preventing the common cold with a garlic supplement: a double-blind, placebo-controlled survey.

https://www.ncbi.nlm.nih.gov/pubmed/11697022

Supplementation with aged garlic extract improves both NK and γδ-T cell function and reduces the severity of cold and flu symptoms: a randomized, double-blind, placebo-controlled nutrition intervention.

https://www.ncbi.nlm.nih.gov/pubmed/22280901

DETOX

Comparison of therapeutic effects of garlic and d-Penicillamine in patients with chronic occupational lead poisoning.

https://www.ncbi.nlm.nih.gov/pubmed/22151785

PAIN

Comparison of effects of ginger, mefenamic acid, and ibuprofen on pain in women with primary dysmenorrhea.

https://www.ncbi.nlm.nih.gov/pubmed/19216660

Daily Ginger Consumption Found to Ease Muscle Pain

http://www.medicalnewstoday.com/articles/189359.php

ARTHRITIS

http://www.arthritis.org/living-with-arthritis/treatments/natural/supplements-herbs/guide/turmeric.php

INFECTIONS

https://www.ncbi.nlm.nih.gov/pubmed/18814211

https://www.ncbi.nlm.nih.gov/pubmed/18814211

https://www.ncbi.nlm.nih.gov/pubmed/23123794

DIABETES & BLOOD SUGAR

https://www.ncbi.nlm.nih.gov/pmc/articles/PMC4277626/

NEUROPROTECTIVE PROPERTIES

http://www.eurekaselect.com/76132

http://www.nature.com/articles/srep38846

http://articles.mercola.com/sites/articles/archive/2013/07/08/-vs-drugs-for-parkinsons.aspx

http://www.sciencedirect.com/science/article/pii/S1357272508002550

TURMERIC AND CIRCULATION

https://www.multivitaminguide.org/blog/-benefits-unclogs-arteries-improves-blood-circulation/

ANTI-INFLAMMATORY

https://www.ncbi.nlm.nih.gov/pubmed/19594223

https://www.ncbi.nlm.nih.gov/pubmed/12676044

CANCER STATISTICS

Cancer Facts & Figures 2017

https://www.cancer.org/research/cancer-facts-statistics/all-cancer-facts-figures/cancer-facts-figures-2017.html

Worldwide cancer statistics

http://www.cancerresearchuk.org/health-professional/cancer-statistics/worldwide-cancer

Economic impact of cancer

http://news.cancerconnect.com/worldwide-cancer-has-biggest-economic-impact-of-any-cause-of-death/

International Agency for Reseach on Cancer – Latest Global Cancer data dated 12 September, 2018

http://www.iarc.fr/en/media-centre/pr/2018/pdfs/pr263_E.pdf

Appendix II: Complete Nutritional Profile for Turmeric, Ginger, & Garlic

Turmeric

Nutrient Data for Turmeric Powder (source USFDA)

Nutrient	1 tsp = 3.0g	1 tbsp = 9.4g
Proximates		
Water	390mg	1.21g
Energy	9kcal	29kcal
Protein	290mg	910mg
Total lipid (fat)	100mg	310mg
Carbohydrate	2.01g	6.31g
Total dietary Fiber	700mg	2100mg
Total Sugars	100mg	300mg
Minerals		
Calcium, Ca	5mg	16mg
Iron, Fe	1.65mg	5.17mg
Magnesium, Mg	6mg	20mg
Phosphorus, P	9mg	28
Potassium, K	62mg	196
Sodium, Na	1mg	3
Zinc, Zn	0.14mg	0.42
Vitamins		
Vitamin C, total ascorbic acid	0	0.1mg
Thiamin	0.002mg	0.005mg
Riboflavin	0.004mg	0.014mg
Niacin	0.041mg	0.127mg

Cancer Prevention

Vitamin B-6	0.003mg	0.01mg
Folate, DFE	1ug	2ug
Vitamin B-12	0	0
Vitamin A, RAE	0	0
Vitamin A, IU	0	0
Vitamin E (alpha-tocopherol)	0.13mg	0.42mg
Vitamin D (D2 + D3)	0	0
Vitamin D	0	0
Vitamin K (phylloquinone)	0.4ug	1.3ug
Lipids		
Fatty acids, total saturated	55mg	173mg
Fatty acids, total monounsaturated	13mg	42mg
Fatty acids, total polyunsaturated	23mg	71mg
Fatty acids, total trans	2mg	5mg
Cholesterol	0	0
Other		
Caffeine	0	0
Alcohol	0	0

Ginger

Nutrient data for Ginger root, raw (source USDA)

Nutrient	1 tsp = 2.0g	0.25 cup slices (1" dia) = 24.0g	5.0 slices (1" dia) = 11.0g
Proximates			
Water	1.58g	18.93g	8.68
Energy	2kcal	19kcal	9
Protein	40mg	440mg	0.2
Total lipid (fat)	10mg	180mg	0.08
Carbohydrate, by difference	360mg	4.26g	1.95
Fiber, total dietary	40mg	500mg	200mg
Sugars, total	30mg	410mg	190mg
Minerals			
Calcium, Ca	0.4mg	4mg	2mg
Iron, Fe	10ug	140ug	70ug
Magnesium, Mg	1mg	10mg	5mg
Phosphorus, P	1mg	8mg	4mg
Potassium, K	8mg	100mg	46mg
Sodium, Na	0.2mg	3mg	1mg
Zinc, Zn	10ug	80ug	40ug
Vitamins			
Vitamin C, total ascorbic acid	100ug	1.2mg	600ug
Thiamin	0.6ug	6ug	3ug
Riboflavin	1ug	8ug	4ug
Niacin	15ug	180ug	83ug
Vitamin B-6	3ug	38ug	18ug
Folate, DFE	0.2ug	3ug	1ug
Vitamin B-12	0	0	0
Vitamin A, RAE	0	0	0

Cancer Prevention

Vitamin A, IU	0	0	0
Vitamin E (alpha-tocopherol)	10ug	60ug	30ug
Vitamin D (D2 + D3)	0	0	0
Vitamin D	0	0	0
Vitamin K (phylloquinone)	0	0	0
Lipids			
Fatty acids, total saturated	4mg	49mg	22ug
Fatty acids, total monounsaturated	3mg	37mg	17ug
Fatty acids, total polyunsaturated	3mg	37mg	17ug
Fatty acids, total trans	0	0	0
Cholesterol	0	0	0
Other			
Caffeine	0	0	0

Garlic

The detailed nutrition chart is below. Source USDA.

Nutrient	1 tsp = 2.8g	1 clove = 3.0g	3.0 cloves = 9.0g
Proximates			
Water	1.64g	1.76g	5.27g
Energy	4kcal	4kcal	13kcal
Protein	0.18g	0.19g	0.57g
Total lipid (fat)	0.01g	0.01g	0.04g
Carbohydrate, by difference	0.93g	0.99g	2.98g
Fiber, total dietary	0.1g	0.1g	0.2g
Sugars, total	0.03g	0.03g	0.09g
Minerals			
Calcium, Ca	5mg	5mg	16mg
Iron, Fe	0.05mg	0.05mg	0.15mg
Magnesium, Mg	1mg	1mg	2mg
Phosphorus, P	4mg	5mg	14mg
Potassium, K	11mg	12mg	36mg
Sodium, Na	1mg	1mg	2mg
Zinc, Zn	0.03mg	0.03mg	0.1mg
Vitamins			
Vitamin C, total ascorbic acid	0.9mg	0.9mg	2.8mg
Thiamin	0.006mg	0.006mg	0.018mg
Riboflavin	0.003mg	0.003mg	0.01mg
Niacin	0.02mg	0.021mg	0.063mg
Vitamin B-6	0.035mg	0.037mg	0.111mg
Folate, DFE	0ug	0ug	0ug
Vitamin B-12	0ug	0ug	0ug
Vitamin A, RAE	0ug	0ug	0ug
Vitamin A, IU	0ug	0ug	1miu

Cancer Prevention

Vitamin E (alpha-tocopherol)	0mg	0mg	0.01mg
Vitamin D (D2 + D3)	0ug	0ug	0ug
Vitamin D	0IU	0IU	0IU
Vitamin K (phylloquinone)	0ug	0.1ug	0.2ug
Lipids			
Fatty acids, total saturated	0.002g	0.003g	0.008g
Fatty acids, total monounsaturated	0g	0g	0.001g
Fatty acids, total polyunsaturated	0.007g	0.007g	0.022g
Fatty acids, total trans	0g	0g	0g
Cholesterol	0mg	0mg	0mg
Amino Acids			
Other			
Caffeine	0mg	0mg	0mg

APPENDIX III. HOME REMEDIES USING GINGER, GARLIC AND TURMERIC

Besides their anti-cancer properties and many other health benefits, turmeric, garlic, and ginger have been used in many home remedies. Some of them are listed below:

GINGER

Nausea: Take a warm cup of ginger tea or ginger soda (see ginger drinks section). The same remedy may be used for morning sickness and motion sickness as well.

Cough: Grate a piece of ginger and boil it in a cup of water with 2-4 crushed peppercorns. Drink lukewarm with optional honey. The same remedy may be used for sore throat and flu as well.

Toothache: Chew a piece of ginger for a few days.

Stomach pain/cramps: Drink ginger tea or ginger ale a couple of times a day.

.

GARLIC

Garlic has been used as a substance against inflections by ancient Egyptians, Greeks, and Romans. They also used it as an aphrodisiac as well as a physical performance enhancing substance.

Cold and flu: Make and drink garlic tea with ginger and lemon 2-3 times a day

Cancer Prevention

Ear infections: Eat raw garlic or consume a garlic drink.

Splinters: Tape/duct tape crushed garlic on the splinter overnight.

Hair loss/thinning: Apply a mixture of garlic oil and coconut oil. Alternatively, rub crushed garlic on the scalp a couple of hours before showering

Toothache: Apply a piece of chopped garlic, bite it gently and hold on the troubled tooth

Sinus infection: Boil 5-7 pieces of garlic and breathe the fumes.

Cough: Roast a piece of garlic and have it with honey.

Athlete's foot: Soak the foot in a bath of warm water containing crushed garlic. Anti-fungal properties in garlic help in curing athlete's foot.

Mosquito repellent: A solution of garlic oil, petroleum jelly, and beeswax can be applied on the skin to prevent mosquito bites.

Cold sores: Hold a piece of crushed garlic directly on the cold sore.

Skin rashes and psoriasis: Apply garlic oil on the affected area.

Cancer Prevention

TURMERIC

Teeth whitening: Sprinkle a bit of turmeric powder on to the store-bought toothpaste before brushing or make your own toothpaste

Healthy skin: Apply a paste made of turmeric mixed with honey or milk or simply water.

Soaps: Add turmeric as part of homemade soaps

Scalp treatment: Add turmeric to warm coconut oil and apply to the scalp and massage it in. Helps prevent scalp issues and improve scalp health.

Temporary tattoos: Turmeric is part of henna to make temporary tattoos.

Making meats safer: Put a teaspoon of turmeric in while washing or cleaning meat. Turmeric kills many of the unsafe microbial organisms in the meat.

Coloring agent: Use it to color Easter eggs, food, and even fabric.

PREVIEW OF OTHER BOOKS IN THIS SERIES

ESSENTIAL SPICES AND HERBS: TURMERIC

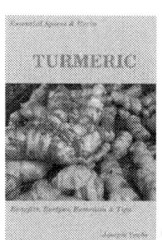

Turmeric is truly a wonder spice. It has anti-inflammatory, anti-oxidant, anti-cancer, and anti-bacterial properties. Find out the amazing benefits of turmeric. Includes many recipes for incorporating turmeric in your daily life.

Turmeric is a spice known to man for thousands of years and has been used for cooking, food preservation, and as a natural remedy for common ailments. This book explains:

- Many health benefits of turmeric including fighting cancer, inflammation, and pain.
- Turmeric as beauty treatments - turmeric masks
- Recipes for teas, smoothies and dishes
- References and links to a number of research studies on the effectiveness of turmeric

Essential Spices and Herbs: Turmeric is a quick read and offers a lot of concise information. A great tool to have in your alternative therapies and healthy lifestyle toolbox!

Cancer Prevention

PREVENTING CANCER

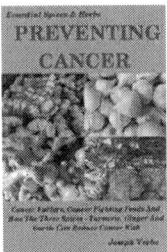

World Health Organization (WHO) estimates more than half of all cancer incidents are preventable.

Cancer is one of the most fearsome diseases to strike mankind. There has been much research into both conventional and alternative therapies for different kinds of cancers. Different cancers require different treatment options and offer a different prognosis. While there has been significant progress in recent times in cancer research towards a cure, there are none available currently. However, more than half of all cancers are likely preventable through modifications in lifestyle and diet.

Preventing Cancer offers a quick insight into cancer-causing factors, foods that fight cancer, and how the three spices, turmeric, ginger and garlic, can not only spice up your food but potentially make all your food into cancer fighting meals. While there are many other herbs and spices that help fight cancer, these three spices work together and complementarily. In addition, the medicinal value of these spices has been proven over thousands of years of use. The book includes:

- Cancer-causing factors and how to avoid them
- Top 12 cancer-fighting foods, the cancers they fight and how to incorporate them into your diet
- Cancer-fighting properties of turmeric, ginger and garlic

Cancer Prevention

- Over 30 recipes including teas, smoothies and other dishes that incorporate these spices
- References and links to many research studies on the effectiveness of these spices.

PREVENTING ALZHEIMER'S

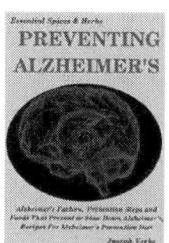

Approximately 50 million people suffer from Alzheimer's worldwide. In the U.S. alone, 5.5 million people have Alzheimer's – about 10 percent of the worldwide Alzheimer's population.

Alzheimer's disease is a progressive brain disorder that damages and eventually destroys brain cells, leading to memory loss, changes in thinking, and other brain functions. While the rate of progressive decline in brain function is slow at the onset, it gets worse with time and age. Brain function decline accelerates, and brain cells eventually die over time. While there has been significant research done to find a cure, currently there is no cure available.

Alzheimer's incidence rate in the U.S. and other western countries is significantly higher than that of the countries in the developing world. Factors such as lifestyle, diet, physical and mental activity, and social engagement play a part in the development and progression of Alzheimer's

In most cases, if you are above the age of 50, plaques and tangles associated with Alzheimer's may have already started forming in your brain. At the age of 65, you have a 10% chance of Alzheimer's and at age 80, the chances are about 50%.

Cancer Prevention

With lifestyle changes, proper diet and exercise (of the mind and body), Alzheimer's is preventable.

In recent times, Alzheimer's is beginning to reach epidemic proportions. The cost of Alzheimer's to the US economy is expected to cross a trillion dollars in 10 years. It is a serious health care issue in many of the western countries as the population age and the life expectancy increase.

At this time, our understanding of what causes Alzheimer's and the ways to treat it is at its infancy. However, we know the factors that affect Alzheimer's and we can use that knowledge to prevent, delay the onset or at least slow down the rate of progression of the disease.

While this book does not present all the answers, it is an attempt to examines the factors affecting Alzheimer's and how to reduce the risk of developing Alzheimer's. A combination of diet and both mental and physical exercise is believed to help in prevention or reducing risk. The book includes:

Discussion on factors in Alzheimer's development

The list of foods that help protect the brain and boost brain health is included in the book:

Over 30 recipes including teas, smoothies, broths, and other dishes that incorporate brain-boosting foods:

References and links to several research studies on Alzheimer's and brain foods.

ALL NATURAL WELLNESS DRINKS

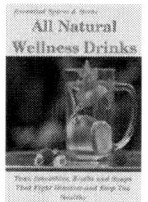

It contains 35 recipes for wellness drinks that include teas, smoothies, soups, and vegan & bone broths. The recipes in this book are unique and combine superfoods, medicinal spices, and herbs. These drinks are anti-cancer, anti-diabetic, ant-aging, heart healthy, anti-inflammatory, and anti-oxidant as well as promote weight loss.

By infusing nature-based nutrients (super fruits and vegetables, spices, and herbs) into drink recipes, we get some amazing wellness drinks that not only replace water loss but nourish the body with vitamins, essential metals, anti-oxidants, and many other nutrients. These drinks may be further enhanced by incorporating spices and herbs along with other superfoods. These drinks not only help heal the body but also enhance the immune system to help prevent many forms of diseases. These drinks may also help rejuvenate the body and delay the aging process. The book also includes suggested wellness drinks for common ailments.

ESSENTIAL SPICES AND HERBS: GINGER

Ginger is a spice known to man for thousands of years and has been used for cooking and as a natural remedy for common ailments. Recent studies have shown that ginger has anti-cancer, anti-inflammatory, and anti-oxidant properties. Ginger helps in reducing muscle pain and is an excellent remedy for nausea. Ginger promotes a healthy digestive system. The book details:

- Many health benefits of ginger including fighting cancer, inflammation, pain and nausea
- Remedies using ginger
- Recipes for teas, smoothies, and other dishes
- References and links to a number of research studies on the effectiveness of ginger

ESSENTIAL SPICES AND HERBS: GARLIC

Garlic is one of the worlds healthiest foods. It helps in maintaining a healthy heart, an excellent remedy for common inflections and has both anti-oxidant and anti-inflammatory properties. It is an excellent food supplement that provides some key vitamins and minerals. This book details the benefits of garlic and describes many easy recipes for incorporating garlic into the diet:

- Many health benefits of garlic including fighting cancer, inflammation, heart health and more
- Remedies using garlic
- Recipes for teas, smoothies, and other dishes
- References and links to a number of research studies on the effectiveness of garlic

ESSENTIAL SPICES AND HERBS: CINNAMON

Cinnamon is an essential spice. It has Anti-diabetic, anti-inflammatory, anti-oxidant, anti-cancer and anti-infections and neuroprotective properties. Cinnamon is a spice known to man for thousands of years and has been used for food preservation, baking, cooking, and as a natural remedy for common ailments. Recent studies have shown that cinnamon has important medicinal properties. This book explains:

- Many health benefits of cinnamon including anti-diabetic, neuroprotective and others.
- Recipes for teas, smoothies, and other dishes
- References and links to a number of research studies on the effectiveness of cinnamon

ANTI-CANCER CURRIES

It is estimated that more than 50% of the cancer incidents are preventable by changing lifestyles, controlling or avoiding cancer-causing factors, or simply eating healthy. There are several foods that are known to have anti-cancer properties either directly or indirectly. Some of these have properties that inhibit cancer cell growth while others have antioxidant and anti-inflammatory properties that contribute to overall health. However, many spices and herbs have direct anti-cancer properties and when one uses anti-cancer spices and herbs in cooking fresh food, there is an immense benefit to be gained. Curry dishes are cooked using many spices that have anti-oxidant, anti-inflammatory, and anti-cancer properties.

This book contains 30 curry recipes that use healthy and anti-cancer ingredients. These recipes are simple and take an average of 20-30 minutes to prepare.

BEGINNERS GUIDE TO COOKING WITH SPICES

Have you ever wondered how to cook with spices? Learn about the many benefits of spices and how to cook with them!

Find out how to start using spices as seasoning and healthy foods. Includes sample recipes,

Beginner's guide to cooking with spices is an introductory book that explains the history, various uses, and their medicinal properties and health benefits. The book details how they may be easily incorporated in everyday cooking. The book will cover the following:

- Health benefits of spices and herbs
- Spice mixes from around the world and their uses
- Tips for cooking with Spices
- Cooking Vegan with Spices
- Cooking Meat and Fish with spices
- Spiced Rice Dishes
- Spicy Soups and Broths

EASY INDIAN INSTANT POT COOKBOOK

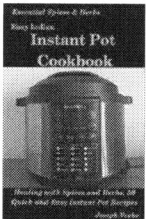

Instant Pot or Electric Pressure Cooker is the most important cooking device in my kitchen. It saves me time, energy, and helps me prepare hassle-free Indian meals all the time.

The Easy Indian Instant Pot Meals contains includes:
- Recipes for 50 Indian dishes
- Tips for cooking with Instant Pot or any electric pressure cooker
- General tips for cooking with spices

FIGHTING THE VIRUS: HOW TO BOOST YOUR BODY'S IMMUNE RESPONSE AND FIGHT VIRUS NATURALLY

What can we do to improve our health and immune response so that our bodies are less prone to viral or bacterial infections? How can we enable our body for a speedy recovery in case of getting such infections?

The answer lies in lifestyle changes that include better hygiene practices, exercise, sleep, and a better diet to keep our body in optimum health. This book is focused on understanding the body's immune system, factors that improve the body's immune response and some natural remedies and recipes. The book contains:
•Overview of the human immune system

Cancer Prevention

- Factors affecting immune response
- Natural substances that fight viral, fungal and bacterial infections
- Recipes that may improve immunity and help speedy recovery
- Supplements that may help improve the immune system
- Scientific studies and references

EASY SPICY EGGS: ALL NATURAL EASY AND SPICY EGG RECIPES

Recipes in this book are not a collection of authentic dishes, but a spicy version of chicken recipes that are easy to make and 100% healthy and flavorful. Ingredients used are mostly natural without any preserved or processed foods.

Most of these recipes include tips and tricks to vary and adapt to your taste of spice level or make with some of the ingredients you like other than the prescribed ingredients in the recipes.

There are about 30 recipes in the book with ideas to make another 30 or even more with the suggestions and notes included with many of the recipes. Cooking does not have to be prescriptive but can be creative. I invite you to try your own variations and apply your creativity to cook dishes that are truly your own.

Cancer Prevention

FOOD FOR THE BRAIN

Nature provides for foods that nourish both the body and the brain. Most often the focus of the diet is physical nourishment, - muscle building, weight loss, energy, athletic performance, and many others. Similar to foods that help the body, there are many foods that help the brain, improve memory and help slow down the aging process. While it is normal to have your physical and mental abilities somewhat slow down with age, diseases such as Alzheimer's, and Parkinson's impact these declines even more. Brain function decline accelerates, and more and more brain cells eventually die over time.

With regular exercises, strength training, practicing martial arts and other physical activities can arrest the physical decline. This book's primary focus is on managing decline in mental and brain function through diet and contains the following:
Characteristics of foods that helps in keeping your brain healthy and young. Brain healthy foods including meats, fruits, vegetables, spices, herbs, and seafood. Supplements to improve memory, cognition and support brain health
Mediterranean diet recipe ideas
DASH diet recipe ideas
Asian diet recipe ideas
Brain boosting supplements and recommendations products and dosage
References

Printed in Great Britain
by Amazon